The SCIENCE-BACKED
MEDITERRANEAN DIET
for Beginners

An Effortless Guide with Simple Meal Plan
To Promote Wellness,Longevity, and Weight Loss

Table of Contents

Introduction

We are what we eat.
- Ludwig Andreas Feuerbach

We live in a unique time in which the relationship between health, prevention, and daily habits is characterized by extreme aspects that, at times, are also paradoxical ones. Food seems to have become a collective obsession: cooking, diets, and nutrition occupy the thoughts of individuals and the spaces of information. In a society of abundance, having forgotten the fear of not having enough food, it seems we hold the solution for well-being and maintaining this condition as long as possible in our lives. Yet, when analyzing epidemiological data, this opportunity seems to elude us, and for a significant portion of the population, food becomes one of the major risk factors for chronic diseases, cancer, cardiovascular diseases, and diabetes.

Something, therefore, is not working: the availability of varied and healthy food does not translate into a better quality of life for everyone, just as the abundance of information we are bombarded with every day does not lead to behaviors that are useful in reducing the risk of illness.

Why? What are the fundamental errors here? On average, too many fats, sugars, and salt are consumed at the table. To this fact, we must add the growing habit of sedentariness, which shifts the energy balance towards a surplus of calories. Economic difficulties for some segments of the population lead to a decrease in meat consumption but, at the same time, to the purchase of low-priced foods, which are not always healthy or of good quality. For the same reason, people frequent fast-food outlets more than restaurants, and give up sports activities and gym memberships, as well as preventive medical check-ups. As if that were not enough, we suffer from increasing stress due to work difficulties, income issues, and social pressure.

For decades now, the Western world has been discussing various containment measures, but the most sustainable and effective solution remains primary prevention. About 80% of cardiovascular diseases and type 2 diabetes, and at least 40% of cancers, can be prevented by improving lifestyle choices (quitting smoking and alcohol, leading a physically active life, and eating a balanced diet). However, every change requires strong motivation and continuous affirmation, a condition in today's climate of mistrust, where half-truths mix with myths, and there's a growing desire for simple solutions and referential figures.

However, to promote individual and collective change with lasting results, it is necessary to act on the deep levers of social behaviors, education, and awareness. And it is on these foundations that this book was written: to offer rigorous, updated, and scientifically-reliable tools for information in the field of nutrition and health. To reclaim that opportunity to act in defense of our health, which we cannot afford to lose.

Premise

Food, diets, healthy eating... Why so much interest in what we bring to the table?
Without food, we cannot live. Food provides all the substances that allow our body to work efficiently and all the energy needed to carry out daily activities. Food is necessary for children to grow, for young people to play and study, for expectant mothers to nourish the coming baby, for adults to work and enjoy their leisure time, and for the elderly to age well. This is the primary reason why it is important to know and take care of what we put on our plate. However, food can also make us sick and, in some cases, even lead to death.

Today, almost one billion people worldwide suffer from hunger, and due to the lack of food, many children exhibit developmental problems. On the other hand, over 2 billion people are obese or overweight, and these conditions—undeniably also linked to improper diet—are at the root of many severe pathologies. The World Health Organization (WHO) estimates that about 33 million deaths each year are related to excessive food intake. With the right diet, at least 30% of cancers can be prevented, according to the World Cancer Research Fund (WCRF), along with a significant percentage of those chronic diseases that represent the main burden of so-called developed countries: diabetes, hypertension, cardiovascular diseases in general, strokes, but also osteoporosis and neurodegenerative diseases such as some dementias.
Choosing the right food means living well and longer.

Do we really need another book on food? What else is there to say?
Everyone talks about food these days: from food bloggers to chefs, from expert nutritionists to celebrities who share the diet they are following. At first glance, this might seem like an ideal scenario, given the enormous amount of information that reaches our homes, but we must not forget that talking about nutrition is not simple, especially if one tries to understand the links between what is put on the plate and health, and if one wants to choose the right foods to stay in shape and prevent diseases based on scientific evidence rather than mere common sense, which is often misleading.

Researchers around the world continue their work tirelessly, and as a result, knowledge about the food-health link is constantly evolving.

In this sense, a current, updated book based solely on data from scientific research and not on trends or dubious news aims to inform while also to focusing on some new aspects of nutrition science, such as the close connection between food and happiness, between food and the future, in the awareness that what we put on our plate influences our health in a holistic way as well as the health of the planet.

The Science-Backed

When discussing the relationship between diet and health, one's immediate thought often goes to which foods should be brought to the table daily and which ones should be avoided. In other instances, the discussion may revolve more generally around the concept of a diet or a healthy eating plan. Studying the impact a single food item has on health is possible (and undoubtedly useful to understand the role that food plays in prevention and maintaining good health), but it is important to emphasize that the ultimate effect of food on the body never depends on a single food item or nutrient. Instead, it results from the combination of foods consumed. For this reason, experts primarily study diets and develop specific ones for certain diseases like hypertension or diabetes.

However, caution is advised when choosing a diet to follow: many "trendy" diets lack scientific foundation and can even harm health.

Nutrition experts who formulate guidelines and recommendations on what to consume to maintain health use various approaches to achieve their goal. Each approach is logically grounded and explores the food-health relationship from a specific perspective.

After all, the modern science of nutrition is actually quite young: the first vitamins were chemically isolated in the early 1900s, which kickstarted the study of individual nutrients found in foods and their effects on health.

It was only in the new millennium that the impact of diet on non-communicable diseases, including cancers, began to be evaluated more systematically. Today, the scientific community is convinced that it's not the individual nutrients within a food item but rather the foods themselves in their entirety—and their combination in daily meals—that truly influence the risk of developing diseases.

It is within this context that we find the Mediterranean diet. As we will see shortly, its effectiveness is not based on calorie counting or the active principles of each ingredient. Instead, it balances diet and lifestyle by considering health as the outcome of all environmental components in which an individual lives: food, physical activity, relationships, and much more.

The Origins of the Mediterranean Diet

Declared an Intangible Cultural Heritage of Humanity by UNESCO in 2010, the Mediterranean diet, as it is defined, is considered by most experts to be one of the healthiest and simplest diets to maintain over the long term. In reality, it is not a single diet but rather a set of eating habits and traditions typical of the Mediterranean area, enriched with nuances depending on the geographical and cultural context.

Some believe the origin of the Mediterranean Diet is as ancient as agriculture itself. It began 10,000 years ago in the Neolithic period when the Sumerians learned to cultivate, and it spread to the countries along the Mediterranean through the Phoenicians. It was the Greeks who gave it the shape that has largely been passed down to us, with the classic trio: wheat, olive oil, and wine.

The Insights of Ancel Keys

The true "mystique" of the Mediterranean Diet originated in the early 1950s when an American researcher named Ancel Keys drew international attention to the low rates of heart disease in some populations of the Mediterranean area.

Born in 1904, Ancel Keys is known for uncovering the modern epidemiology of cardiovascular diseases and for formulating, on behalf of the U.S. Department of Defense, balanced meals for combat soldiers still known as "K rations," from the initial of his last name. Alongside his studies on the correlation between diet, cholesterol levels, and the risk of cardiovascular diseases, Keys and his wife Margaret, a nutritionist and culinary scholar, wrote two widely distributed books, including "Eat Well and Stay Well, the Mediterranean Way." With these works, they earned the great merit of being the first to describe the value of the Mediterranean Diet in the Anglo-Saxon world, not only from a health perspective but also for its gastronomic significance.

Keys spent much of his life in Italy. He landed in Salerno in 1945 with the Fifth Army in the territory of Battipaglia and noticed that cardiovascular diseases were very limited in that area, although prevalent in the United States. In particular, among the population of Cilento, the incidence of what are today called "diseases of affluence" (atherosclerosis, hypertension, diabetes, etc.) was notably low.

In the immediate post-war period, Keys became interested in better understanding the association between diet and cardiovascular diseases: American businessmen, presumably the best-fed people, had high rates of heart disease, while in post-war Europe, rates of cardiovascular diseases had sharply decreased, coinciding with a drastic reduction in food availability. Postulating a correlation between cholesterol levels and cardiovascular diseases, in 1948 Keys launched the first prospective study related to cardiovascular diseases, which lasted 15 years, on a group of businessmen from Minnesota. It showed that at blood cholesterol levels above 260, the risk of contracting cardiovascular diseases within a few years was four to six times greater compared to those who had a cholesterol level below 200-220.

The Seven Countries Study

To scientifically demonstrate the health benefits of the Mediterranean diet, Ancel Keys embarked on the observational study later known as the "Seven Countries Study," which compared the diets of seven countries (United States, Italy, Finland, Greece, Yugoslavia, Netherlands, and Japan) to assess their benefits and critical points in terms of cardiovascular health.

The results were clear: the further one deviated from Mediterranean dietary patterns, the higher the incidence of cardiovascular diseases. Recent scientific literature can help us hypothesize why the Mediterranean diet has a protective effect on health: firstly, this dietary style includes the consumption of low calorie density foods such as vegetables, fruits, cereals, and legumes, which also provide a fiber intake that protects against many chronic and degenerative diseases; moreover, numerous positive biological activities for our organism have been found in compounds present almost exclusively in plant-based foods.

There is now ample scientific evidence, as we will see later, of the effectiveness of this nutritional model not only in preventing cardiovascular diseases but also in protecting against diseases such as cancer, obesity, and diabetes. Moreover, the Mediterranean diet reduces the risk of osteoporosis and cognitive problems while also protecting against the development of many types of cancer, including breast, colorectal, prostate, stomach, and liver cancer. Finally, but no less importantly, there are studies that explain how the Mediterranean diet also has a positive impact on mood disorders, significantly reducing the risk of depression.

The Relevance of the Mediterranean Diet Today

It is interesting to note that in 1977, when a U.S. Senate Committee presented its report on the health status of American citizens and the need for a prevention campaign that would modify dietary habits in light of the results of the "Seven Countries Study," Italy had already greatly diverged from the virtuous model celebrated by Ancel Keys, with the average consumption of meat, for example, having quadrupled.

Today, even in Mediterranean countries, there is an increasingly widespread diffusion of the typical diet model of the United States, which is gradually modifying the food traditions of many areas of the Western world, including Italy and Greece, and is rapidly spreading even to distant countries such as China or India, which boast food traditions completely different from those of the so-called developed countries.

In summary, this "Western diet" is based on a high consumption of saturated fats and refined sugars and a very low consumption of fiber because fruits and vegetables are very scarce on the tables.

What are the health risks of following a Western diet? Overweight and obesity, cardiovascular diseases, hypertension, metabolic diseases such as type 2 diabetes, inflammatory bowel diseases, and many cancers are just some of the conditions that can arise from following this type of diet on a daily basis. After all, the data are clear: in the United States and most Western countries, chronic diseases related to diet are the leading cause of illness and mortality, a real epidemic that affects in one way or another 50-60% of the adult population of the Western or "Westernized" world. Scientists are also studying new mechanisms underlying the negative impact of this diet on health, and there are increasingly numerous studies demonstrating how Western food is harmful to the proper functioning of the immune system and the microbiota, the community of microorganisms that populate our intestines and help us stay healthy.

Health and Diet

Numerous scientific studies conducted since the time of Ancel Keys to the present have shown that the Mediterranean diet plays an important role in preventing many diseases. The beneficial effects of this dietary pattern are linked to several factors, such as the abundance of low caloric density foods (vegetables, fruits, cereals, and legumes), which help maintain a healthy weight and ensure a fiber intake that protects against the onset of many chronic diseases.

The Mediterranean diet is also characterized by a low content of fats, mostly unsaturated fats, and a high intake of antioxidants, which counteract the harmful effects of free radicals, including the polyphenols in extra virgin olive oil and lycopene in tomatoes. Most studies on the Mediterranean diet and lifestyle have demonstrated its effectiveness in all major health areas:

- Prevention of chronic diseases and inflammation
- Weight loss
- Longevity and successful aging

Let's now look at all its benefits in detail.

Prevention of Chronic Diseases and Inflammation

In the more advanced regions of the world, the main causes of mortality are non-communicable diseases, different from those of bacterial or viral origin, which, fortunately, are decreasing in the Western world thanks to improvements in hygiene and the use of vaccinations. In recent years, it has become increasingly clear that these "affluence diseases" arise precisely because of the Western lifestyle, particularly due to suboptimal dietary habits.

The Western diet has a significant impact on functions, physiology, and cardiovascular pathologies such as myocardial infarction, heart failure, hypertension, etc., and the benefits of adopting a Mediterranean lifestyle in terms of prevention have been scientifically known for many years. In recent decades, the entire world of scientific research has been engaged in studying the impact of diet on the other huge "epidemic" of the richest countries, namely the oncological emergency. Thanks to research, we now know that about a third of cancer cases start to develop from modifiable behaviors and habits, including those we follow at the table, and the protective effect offered by the Mediterranean diet is a certainty also in the field of cancer, although the mechanisms underlying the biological effects and inflammation have not yet been fully clarified.

Cardiovascular Diseases and Metabolic Syndrome

Many studies associate the Mediterranean diet with a reduced risk of developing cardiovascular diseases. Positive effects derive from a set of characteristics of this dietary pattern:

- Low content of saturated fats.
- Abundance of unsaturated fats, such as omega-3 from fish and nuts and oleic acid from extra virgin olive oil.
- Reduced salt consumption in favor of spices and herbs.

These elements help control cholesterol and triglyceride levels, benefiting heart health and preventing conditions such as hypertension. For the same reasons, the Mediterranean diet also proves to be an ally against metabolic syndrome, a set of conditions (obesity, diabetes, arterial hypertension, cholesterol, high triglycerides) that expose us to a high cardiovascular risk.

Obesity and Type 2 Diabetes Mellitus

The Mediterranean diet represents a complete and balanced dietary regime, ideal for those looking to lose weight or maintain it. It is low in fats, most of which are unsaturated, rich in low calorie density foods, provides plenty of fiber that promotes satiety, and—with quantities modulated on one's own needs—is perfect for getting back in shape. Also, it is a varied diet, never monotonous, full of tasty dishes, three important elements for those following a low-calorie regime to lose weight or for those wishing to maintain the weight loss results achieved over the long term.

Despite being rich in carbohydrates in the form of whole grains like bread and pasta, it is advisable even for diabetics. The key lies in selecting slow-release carbohydrates present in whole foods, which help maintain stable blood sugar levels. Sugary foods, on the other hand, which are at the top of the pyramid and whose consumption is suggested to be very limited, rapidly increase blood sugar levels and should be avoided. The presence of fiber in meals, especially soluble ones, can moderate sugar absorption, recommending dishes rich in vegetables instead of simple ones. A proper diet for diabetics must always be personalized by specialists considering various individual factors such as age, weight, and physical activity; however, in general terms, a balanced Mediterranean diet, which is not limited to bread and pasta but includes a wide variety of healthy foods such as fruit, vegetables, legumes, fish, and extra virgin olive oil, promotes a balanced approach to diet and lifestyle, which can be of great help to those suffering from diabetes.

Cancer

Today, we understand that inflammation can facilitate the transformation of normal cells into cancerous ones and support their uncontrolled growth. Another risk factor is undoubtedly linked to body weight control. Excess weight triggers a series of mechanisms—from an increase in inflammation itself to increases in blood sugar and circulating insulin levels—that fuel the development and cellular proliferation in a cancerous direction. The Mediterranean diet, with its ability to help maintain an ideal weight and its famously protective foods, has been proven to protect against the onset of many types of cancer.

Specifically, scientific studies demonstrate its effectiveness in preventing at least 12 types of cancers: oral, stomach, colorectal, breast, pancreatic, gallbladder, liver, ovarian, kidney, esophageal, prostate cancers, as well as cervical and uterine body cancers. The credit for these significant health benefits goes to the richness of antioxidants, which combat cell degeneration caused by free radicals, and the low content of fats (mostly unsaturated, such as the beneficial omega-3 with anti-inflammatory action).

Additionally, the high fiber content improves intestinal transit, ensuring potentially dangerous substances do not remain in contact with the intestine's walls for too long (a risk factor for colorectal cancer). There are also substances with specific anticancer actions present in some vegetables. Among these, glucosinolates from cruciferous vegetables (broccoli, cauliflower) and the sulfur compounds abundant in onions.

The beneficial effects on cancer prevention are also linked to the Mediterranean diet's ability to maintain a healthy microbiota, the complex of microorganisms (bacteria, viruses, fungi, protozoa) that normally colonize our entire body. The most studied microbiota is the intestinal one. A healthy microbiota is crucial for our well-being and is also fundamental for cancer prevention: variations in its composition are indeed associated with the development of many diseases, including cancer. The Mediterranean diet, rich in cereals, fruits, and vegetables high in antioxidants and fiber, creates the ideal "climate" to encourage the proliferation of "good" bacteria and keep the microbiota healthy.

Weight Loss

In the "ranking" of diets, the Mediterranean diet surpasses all others, also claiming the top spot among the best diets for weight loss. Compared to other more "fashionable" eating plans, science shows that the Mediterranean dietary regime, combined with a healthy lifestyle, is the most effective way to ensure lasting weight loss. And, thanks to the reduction of all the risk factors we've just discussed, an overall improvement in health conditions. A study published in the journal Advances in Nutrition suggests that diets promising desired results in a few weeks often lose effectiveness over time, with the risk of worsening the conditions of those who follow them.

This consideration emerges from the conclusions of a review of about 80 revisions and meta-analyses available, analyzing variations in anthropometric parameters (starting with body weight) and cardiometabolic risk factors (total blood cholesterol, LDL, HDL, triglycerides, glucose, insulin, glycated hemoglobin levels, and blood pressure) determined by 11 of the most popular diets. Specifically: low-carb or low-fat diets, high-protein diets, the paleolithic diet, the Zone diet, the vegetarian diet, the Nordic diet, the DASH diet, the Mediterranean diet, and the portfolio diet. The review confirmed the "primacy" of the Mediterranean diet for managing weight and preventing the onset of chronic diseases, first and foremost, type 2 diabetes. Moreover, according to a study published in 2016 in the journal Obesity Reviews, more than 4 in 10 adults have tried to diet at least once in their life, and browsing the pages of the publication, what emerges is that almost all the most fashionable diets can have negative health consequences, without ensuring that the weight loss will continue in the long term.

Many wonder how it is possible to lose weight following the Mediterranean diet where there are no particular restrictions and what scientific evidence supports this correlation. The answer lies in the quality and variety of the foods that make up this diet. Focusing on nutrient-rich foods and moderate portions, listening to the body's hunger and satiety signals, and integrating physical exercise, it's possible to embark on an effective and enjoyable weight loss journey. Weight loss is generally slower and more gradual than with "crash diets," but this makes it more reliable and sustainable.

To achieve optimal results with the Mediterranean diet, if you wish to lose weight, it's important to consider three main aspects, these three pillars form a comprehensive approach to a healthy lifestyle that is both sustainable and beneficial for long-term health and well-being:

1. **EATING HABITS:** Regular meal times and choosing nutritious snacks are essential for maintaining health and managing weight. The practice of waiting 15-20 minutes before taking a second serving can help better gauge fullness, and among the most effective strategies is also the so-called 80% rule or the Hara Hachi Bu principle from Okinawa. In this Japanese island, home to one of the world's longest-lived populations, there's an unwritten rule to eat until you are 80% full. It's a simple concept: eat until you're satisfied, not stuffed. This approach, which is also considered good table manners in Italy—always leaving a little space in your stomach when you leave the table—helps control weight and has significant health benefits, such as developing a keen sense of one's body and fostering an intuitive rather than emotional eating style.

2. **PHYSICAL EXERCISE:** As with any dietary regimen, the Mediterranean diet encourages the integration of regular physical activity to support weight loss and maintain overall good health. Unlike other highly restrictive diets, the Mediterranean diet excels because it does not deprive followers of essential nutrients or the energy needed to safely and healthily engage in physical activity. In terms of exercise choice, the Mediterranean lifestyle encourages finding enjoyable types of movement to ensure greater continuity and long-term sustainability.

3. **HYDRATION:** Drinking plenty of water helps keep the body hydrated, aids digestion, and can prevent episodes of hunger caused by thirst. Proper hydration is a fundamental part of

the Mediterranean lifestyle, complementing the diet and exercise components to support overall health.

These principles, central to the Mediterranean way of life, emphasize the importance of balance, moderation, and enjoyment in one's approach to food and lifestyle. By adopting these habits, individuals can enjoy a range of health benefits, including improved weight management, enhanced physical well-being, and a greater sense of satisfaction and happiness in daily life.

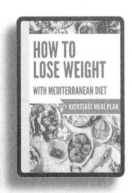

Do you need to lose weight?

To complement the general MEAL PLAN in the book, which does not specifically address weight loss needs, I've also created two variations.

You can download the 1200-calorie plan and the 2000-calorie plan as an additional resource. **On page 155**, you will find all the instructions to access them.

5 Mediterranean Tips

To successfully incorporate the Mediterranean diet into your daily routine, here are five practical tips:

1. Start your day with a fiber-rich breakfast such as whole grains with fruit and Greek yogurt. The abundance of antioxidants and healthy fats, along with high fiber content, promotes good digestion and a prolonged sense of satiety, helping to control appetite and avoid overeating.

2. Prepare healthy snacks to consume throughout the day, like raw vegetables with hummus or a handful of nuts. Light and frequent snacks are a staple of the Mediterranean diet that can provide satisfaction and keep hunger at bay.

3. Experiment with recipes using legumes and whole grains as the main ingredients. Don't fear carbohydrates; they can provide you with good energy. The key is moderation and paying attention to dressings. This means you shouldn't give up on your portion of pasta or other grains, which help you achieve and maintain a good level of satiety, but opt for dressings with raw oil instead of elaborate sauces or gravies.

4. Follow a meal plan, as research suggests that people who plan their meals are generally less likely to develop obesity or overweight. Specifically, losing weight always requires some intentionality, and one way to ensure you firmly adhere to the Mediterranean diet is to dedicate time to meal planning. This avoids reaching lunch or dinner time with few ideas, the rush to eat something, and a refrigerator that's empty or filled with unsuitable foods.

5. Try to eat meals in company, valuing the mealtime as an opportunity for sharing and pleasure.
In conclusion, one of the most appreciated aspects of the Mediterranean diet is its sustainability over time. By not imposing severe restrictions, it allows you to enjoy food and the conviviality of meals without giving up the pleasure of eating. The variety of foods proposed ensures a wide range of essential nutrients and promotes a balanced relationship with food. This non-punitive approach, which doesn't demonize any food but rather encourages moderate and mindful consumption, becomes the key to healthy and lasting weight loss while promoting physical health and psychological well-being.

Pregnancy

The Mediterranean diet is also recommended during pregnancy as a healthy eating regimen. It helps to manage weight gain, protecting the expectant mother from the risk of metabolic complications, including gestational diabetes, which can have serious consequences for both the mother's and the baby's health.

Following this dietary regimen can also be beneficial for women entering pregnancy with pre-existing issues like:

- obesity,
- chronic hypertension,
- elevated lipid levels.

Longevity and Successful Aging

In recent decades, the secret to a long and prosperous life seems to have been unveiled through extensive studies on the Mediterranean diet, which, as numerous studies and scientific research attest, is capable of promoting longevity and "successful aging."

A recent study conducted in Italy by the NFI (Nutrition Foundation of Italy), for example, examined the link between adherence to the Mediterranean diet and various aspects of health in the elderly, including mental health, cognitive status, and quality of life. The results showed that those who most faithfully followed this diet were less likely to experience cognitive decline and depressive symptoms and enjoyed a better quality of life. These benefits are attributed to the diet's rich composition of essential nutrients, antioxidants, and healthy fats, which together play a key role in modulating inflammatory and oxidative processes, positively influencing both physical and mental health.

Furthermore, adherence to the Mediterranean diet has been linked, as we have already seen, to a reduction in the risk of developing chronic diseases such as cardiovascular diseases, type 2 diabetes, and certain forms of cancer. The presence of omega-3 fatty acids, particularly from fish consumption (including salmon, herring, sardines, and bluefish in general), plays a crucial role in preventing inflammation and promoting brain health, reducing the risk of cognitive decline.

The Mediterranean lifestyle, which combines a balanced diet with healthy physical exercise, further amplifies health benefits, helping to maintain ideal body weight, strengthen muscles and bones, improve mobility and flexibility; all essential aspects for successful aging.

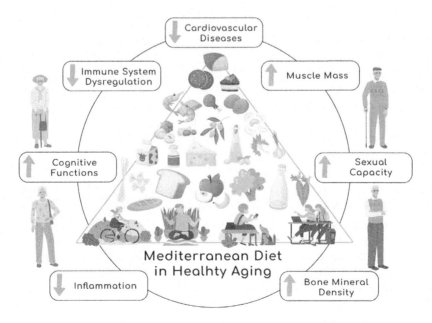

Mediterranean Diet
in Healhty Aging

Thus, in an era where life expectancy continues to rise, adopting the Mediterranean diet can be the foundation on which to build a path to slow, healthy, and happy aging. Beyond nutrition and physical activity aspects, the Mediterranean diet also emphasizes the importance of a balanced approach to life, including proper rest and stress management, moderation in food consumption, and attention to the variety and seasonality of ingredients... encouraging a harmonious relationship with food, where it is not only a source of nutrition but also of pleasure and sharing.

Depressive States

The Mediterranean diet emerges as a powerful ally against depression, promoting a significant improvement in mental well-being. This dietary model is distinguished by its ability to reduce inflammation, a factor often linked to depressive disorders. Two Australian studies have demonstrated how adopting this diet leads to a clear improvement in depressive symptoms, offering a revolutionary perspective in treating this condition.

The approach used in the studies involved dividing participants suffering from depression into two groups: the first received dietary counseling aimed at promoting the adoption of the Mediterranean diet, while the other group participated in social support sessions. Interestingly, unlike conventional therapies, the group following the Mediterranean dietary regime showed significant improvements, as evidenced by depression rating scales. These results underline how a healthy diet can not only prevent depression but can actually positively influence its course. The Mediterranean diet, in particular, is based on "brain-friendly" foods, such as whole grains, fruits, vegetables, and fish, while reducing the consumption of harmful foods like refined cereals or fried, sugary, and processed foods.

The importance of an anti-inflammatory diet, rich in B vitamins and folates, lies in its ability to improve neuroplasticity, the brain's ability to form new neural connections, thus favoring recovery from depression. Whole and natural foods are fundamental for maintaining optimal health of the intestinal microbiota, whose balance directly affects overall well-being and, in particular, mental health, with observable changes just two or three weeks after adoption.

The positive impact on the microbiota, in turn, has the power to influence mood and psychological well-being, although the exact time needed to observe an improvement in mood remains to be determined.

The importance of a balanced diet thus goes beyond simple nutrition, deeply impacting mental health and offering a real opportunity for improvement for those suffering from depression. Encouraging adherence to the Mediterranean diet represents not just a prevention strategy but also a potential therapeutic intervention, opening new paths for a more holistic approach to mental health.

Aging and Cognitive Decline

A study coordinated by researchers from Columbia University in New York and published in the journal Archives of Neurology has found that the Mediterranean diet also helps prevent cognitive decline, through a protective action on the brain system. Discussing the Mediterranean diet as an elixir of long life is no longer far-fetched, confirmed by the results of a study conducted by the University of Gothenburg known as the "H70 Study."

The investigation, which began 40 years ago, was conducted by comparing a group of 70-year-olds who followed a diet based on the Mediterranean model with a peer group whose diet was rich in animal products. It was found that people who follow a diet based on the Mediterranean model have a 20% higher chance of living longer, on average by two to three years, compared to those who primarily consume meat and proteins.

Moreover, the Mediterranean diet is confirmed as an effective prevention tool against neurodegenerative diseases such as Alzheimer's and Parkinson's. This dietary regimen, rich in antioxidants, omega-3 fatty acids, and fiber, plays a key role in neuroprotection by combating inflammation and oxidative stress, mechanisms at the heart of neurodegeneration.

The abundant amount of fiber introduced with a diet strongly based on plant products and cereals promotes a balanced gut microbiota, essential for brain health, producing compounds that counteract inflammation. The correct intake of nutrients that the Mediterranean diet promotes also supports weight control, minimizing further risk factors for Alzheimer's and Parkinson's, namely overweight and obesity.

Completing the beneficial framework are the antioxidants and healthy fats that prevent cellular alterations and promote neural well-being. This comprehensive approach not only underscores the significant impact of the Mediterranean diet on physical health but also highlights its profound implications for mental and cognitive health, offering a promising avenue for the prevention and management of cognitive decline and neurodegenerative diseases.

Decline in Bone mass and Osteoporosis

Diet is increasingly recognized as a modifiable factor in bone and muscle health. The latest discovery regarding osteoporosis in affected individuals highlights that a diet rich in fruits, vegetables, whole grains, fish, and extra virgin olive oil can reduce bone mass loss. The Mediterranean diet, characterized by high consumption of these foods, demonstrated positive effects in a study conducted on over a thousand elderly individuals aged 65 to 79 years across five European countries. Published in the American Journal of Clinical Nutrition, the findings indicate that while the diet does not affect individuals with normal bone density values, it has a significant impact on those with osteoporosis, particularly in the femoral neck, a common site for fractures in old age.

Interestingly, the authors of the study exclude the benefits being due to vitamin D supplementation, suggesting instead a potential protective role of phenolic compounds present in extra virgin olive oil. These compounds could promote the maturation of osteoblasts and the deposition of calcium, which is crucial in pathologies like osteoporosis and sarcopenia that increase frailty and susceptibility to fractures, morbidity, and mortality.

This insight underscores the importance of dietary choices in managing and potentially mitigating the effects of age-related bone density loss. The Mediterranean diet, with its emphasis on nutrient-rich, natural foods, and healthy fats, provides a comprehensive approach to supporting bone and muscle health, thereby contributing to a reduction in the risk of osteoporosis-related complications. Such findings highlight the need for further research into the specific components of the diet that confer these benefits, as well as the mechanisms by which they operate, offering hope for non-pharmacological interventions in the management of osteoporosis and improving the quality of life for the elderly.

HEALTH BENEFITS ACROSS THE LIFE CYCLE
EATING A MEDITERRANEAN DIET IS LINKED WITH...

Lower risk of child asthma and wheeze	Improved odds of a successful pregnancy with IVF in women	Significantly less plaque buildup in arteries	Improvement in silent reflux (just as effective as medication)	38% lower risk of frailty in older adults (60+)
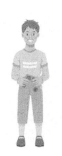	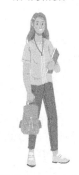	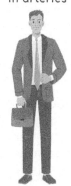	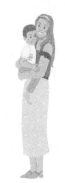	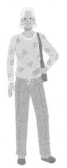
Lower odds of having ADHD in kids	30% lower risk of hearth disease and significantly lower risk of stroke in high-risk	Less need for multiple medications	Lower risk of high plessure, unhealthy cholesterol levels, and diabetes	Improved cognitive performance - particularly memory - and lower dementia rates

Getting Started

How does the Mediterranean diet work?

More than just a diet in its countries of origin, the Mediterranean diet represents a lifestyle, a holistic approach to food considered as a fundamental element of life, a social celebration, and an occasion to gather with friends and family. This dietary pattern transcends the mere notion of a temporary or restrictive diet regimen; the Mediterranean diet isn't a 30-day fast or a 10-day no-carb diet, it's a healthy way of living that you can stick to for the rest of your life. In fact, hundreds of millions of people already eat this way. Diets are usually short-lived, or very specific, and unsustainable in the long run. The Mediterranean style, however, is a healthy way of living whose flexibility allows easy integration of its habits, promoting the well-being of the entire family for a lifetime.

The Mediterranean diet Pyramid

The recommendations for healthy eating issued by various scientific societies may vary slightly and are generally the result of years of research. They are often represented in simple and intuitive graphic forms, and the most famous of these models is undoubtedly the food pyramid, first proposed in 1992 by experts from the U.S. Department of Agriculture to explain how often to consume foods. Over the years, the pyramid has been modified several times to keep pace with new medical discoveries and to meet the needs of different populations (elderly, children, etc.) and different cultural contexts.

Today's food pyramid is structured in several tiers, where different food groups are arranged in a hierarchical manner, each characterized by a different nutrient content and with their recommended portion sizes on a daily or weekly basis. Within the same food group, it's very important to vary the choice and differentiate the ingredients to achieve as varied and complete a diet as possible. At the base of the pyramid, there are plant-based foods that are characteristic of the "Mediterranean diet" for their abundance of non-energetic nutrients (vitamins, minerals, water) and protective compounds (fiber and phytochemicals: bioactive compounds of plant origin). Moving up the pyramid, there are foods with higher energy density that should be consumed in smaller quantities.

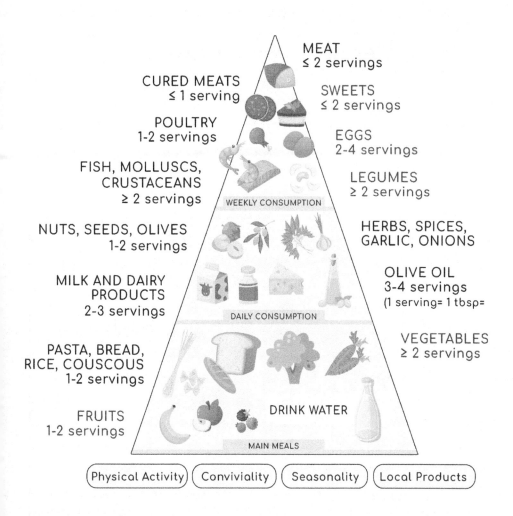

MEAT
≤ 2 servings

CURED MEATS
≤ 1 serving

SWEETS
≤ 2 servings

POULTRY
1-2 servings

EGGS
2-4 servings

FISH, MOLLUSCS,
CRUSTACEANS
≥ 2 servings

LEGUMES
≥ 2 servings

WEEKLY CONSUMPTION

NUTS, SEEDS, OLIVES
1-2 servings

HERBS, SPICES,
GARLIC, ONIONS

MILK AND DAIRY
PRODUCTS
2-3 servings

OLIVE OIL
3-4 servings
(1 serving= 1 tbsp=

DAILY CONSUMPTION

PASTA, BREAD,
RICE, COUSCOUS
1-2 servings

VEGETABLES
≥ 2 servings

FRUITS
1-2 servings

DRINK WATER

MAIN MEALS

(Physical Activity) (Conviviality) (Seasonality) (Local Products)

For those seeking a more immediate, albeit less precise, representation, they can follow the "Healthy Eating Plate" model developed by the Harvard School of Public Health, which indicates what the best composition of each meal should be. In summary, half of the plate should consist of vegetables and fruit (with a preference for vegetables less rich in sugars compared to fruit), the other half should equally represent whole grains and healthy proteins (from fish, legumes, and poultry).

HEALTHY EATING PLATE

The more vegetables and variety, the better! Potatoes and French fries don't count as vegetables.

Eat different varieties of whole grains (whole grain bread, whole grain pasta and whole grain rice). Limit refined cereals (white rice and white bread)

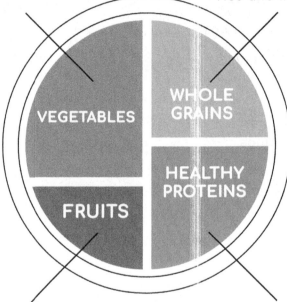

VEGETABLES

WHOLE GRAINS

FRUITS

HEALTHY PROTEINS

Eat plenty of fruit, of all colors.

Choose fish, poultry, legumes and oilseeds; limit red meat and cheese; avoid bacon, cold cuts and other processed meats.

Use healthy oils (such as olive oil and canola oil) for cooking and dressing. Limit butter. Avoid trans fats.

Drink water, tea or coffee (with little or no sugar). Limit milk and dairy products (1-2 servings per day) and fruit juices (1 small glass per day). Avoid sugary drinks.

As it becomes clear, the Mediterranean Pyramid does not provide actual caloric indications as most other diets tend to do, nor is it absolutely restrictive regarding particular food groups. The guidelines of this dietary plan are rather related to the consumption frequency of each ingredient or food group.

It's noteworthy that the entire pyramid is built on a solid foundation of daily physical activity, conviviality, and sharing opportunities, which we will explore in the final chapters of the book and which indeed make the Mediterranean diet more akin to a true lifestyle rather than a dietary regimen.

Moreover, the quality of the raw materials used in cooking is also an essential element for understanding the health role of a traditional diet that focuses on the seasonality of plant ingredients.

Finally, something that is discussed less frequently but is important to consider is that the effectiveness of this diet does not reside solely in the quality of the individual foods but also in the synergies between them. Learning to cook Mediterranean means learning the typical combinations of various ingredients according to the traditional model, to enjoy their maximum benefits. Particularly effective combinations include:

- Bread, pasta, and legumes dressed with oil;
- Wild salads dressed with oil and vinegar;
- Roasted vegetables, treated with vinegar, oil, and herbs;
- Fish fried in oil after flouring;
- Extensive use of fresh garlic and onion;
- Extensive use of tomato, including concentrated or dehydrated.

The effect of these combinations is still little known; however, we understand that consuming vegetables with oil enhances the assimilation of water-insoluble active substances. The roasting of meats can lead to the formation of pro-oxidant and potentially carcinogenic substances, while the roasting or frying of vegetable products results in the formation of antioxidants and bacteriostatic substances. Similarly, the prolonged heating used to concentrate tomato juice traditionally, when preparing one of the most classic dishes of Italian Mediterranean cuisine: pasta with tomato sauce.

Weekly Portions

As mentioned, the Mediterranean diet isn't based on calorie counting but rather on the balance of various food groups within the plate and throughout the week. The unit of measure used in the food pyramid and by nutritionists formulating Mediterranean-type diet plans is the commonly known servings.

Here are the guidelines for the portions of various foods to be consumed on a daily or weekly basis:

- For fruits and vegetables, 4-5 servings per day are recommended, with a weekly consumption of 12 servings of fruit and 18 servings of vegetables. A fruit serving should weigh about 5.3 oz, corresponding to a medium/large fruit (like apples, pears, oranges, peaches, or similar) or two/three pieces in the case of mandarins, plums, apricots, or other small fruits.

- For pasta and rice, the reference portion is 3 oz for dry pasta and 4 oz for fresh egg pasta. It's advised to have a pasta serving per day, with up to a maximum of 12 servings a week, including pasta and rice, preferably whole grains.

- For legumes, the reference portion is about 1 oz (dry) or 3.5 oz (fresh); with a recommended consumption of 2-3 servings a week.

- Fish, the reference portion is about 5.3 oz, with a recommended weekly consumption of at least 2-3 servings.

- For eggs, the reference portion is one egg, with a recommendation to consume a maximum of 2-3 eggs a week.

- For meat, the reference portion is 3.5 oz of meat (raw), with a recommendation to eat a maximum of 3-4 servings a week, thus not every day, preferring white meats (chicken, rabbit, turkey) instead.

- For processed meats, the reference portion corresponds to 1.7 oz, about 3 slices of ham, with a recommended consumption of up to a maximum of 2 servings weekly, so not every day!

- For milk, the reference portion corresponds to 1/2 cup of skim milk or yogurt. The recommendation is 1-2 servings per day, with a weekly consumption of a maximum of 18 servings.

- For cheeses, the reference portion is 1.7 oz for aged cheese and 3.5 oz for fresh cheese. It's advised to consume a maximum of 2 servings a week.

- For dressings, preferably extra virgin olive oil, the reference portion is 2 tsp, with 3-4 portions recommended per day, totaling 24 portions a week.

In this distribution, it's clear that fruits and vegetables should dominate the diet, followed by cereals, especially whole grains. The reference to portions is necessary to avoid exceeding quantities, i.e., eating less and better. Additionally, it's very important to reduce the amount of salt, use herbs and spices as flavorings, eliminate sugary beverages, and consume at least half of the grains as whole ones.

Water also has a place within the pyramid and is found at the base, among the most important groups. The recommended amount of water for an adult is at least 1.5-2 liters a day.

Food Groups and Active Ingredients

Following the Mediterranean diet means ensuring a balanced intake according to a dietary pattern that provides your body with:

- Moderate amounts of proteins, predominantly of plant origin.
- Low glycemic index carbohydrates, with almost no simple sugars.
- A high ratio of monounsaturated to saturated fatty acids.
- A large amount of antioxidants (beta-carotene, tocopherols, vitamins C and E, polyphenols).
- An abundance of calcium, magnesium, and potassium, with low amounts of sodium.

Energy is derived from macronutrients (carbohydrates, proteins, and fats) and should be distributed as follows to be considered a "balanced" diet:

- 45–60% from carbohydrates, predominantly complex (like cereal starches).
- 10–12% from proteins, favoring plant sources, fish, and lean white meats.
- 20–35% from fats, with a percentage of saturated fats (mostly found in almost all animal products except fish) under 10%.

But from which food groups do these nutrients come?

Cereals and Byproducts

The Mediterranean diet recommends the intake of 1-2 servings of cereals per day. This group includes well-known carbohydrates, such as pasta, rice, and breakfast cereals, but also many other traditional cereals, like barley, spelt, and millet. Ideally, whole or unrefined grains should be consumed to preserve their nutritional value in terms of vitamins, minerals, essential fatty acids, and fibers, which represent the real wealth of cereals.

Carbohydrates are the main source of readily-available energy. They are distinguished into simple, quickly-assimilated ones, and complex ones. Simple carbohydrates are found in fruit, milk, jam, honey, sugar, and give a sweet flavor to foods; complex carbohydrates, on the other hand, are present in pasta, rice, potatoes, and legumes.

If consumed in excess, carbohydrates can turn into fats, but if taken in insufficient amounts, they force the body to convert the proteins from meat into energy, straining the body and forcing it to compensate in an unhealthy way.

Healthy eating guidelines suggest that in a well-composed and balanced diet, 45-60% of the calories should come from carbohydrates, three-quarters of which should be in the form of complex carbohydrates, and the remaining quarter as simple ones.

The importance of carbohydrates comes from the fact that they are easily absorbed and utilized by the body, ensuring cells the necessary supply of glucose and energy.

Maintaining a correct balance between calories consumed and expended is important. A diet rich in carbohydrates makes us less inclined to accumulate fat compared to one low in carbohydrates but rich in lipids. Carbohydrates satisfy quickly, and, particularly fiber-rich foods are relatively bulky and satisfying.

Pasta: Friend or Foe?

Whether it's fusilli, penne, or simple spaghetti, some people just can't resist a plate of pasta. Perhaps it's due to the presence of tryptophan, an amino acid that the body uses to synthesize mood-boosting hormones and neurotransmitters. Or maybe it's the savory taste known as "umami," which is especially pronounced when paired with tomato sauce and a sprinkle of cheese, a simple and beloved Italian topping rich in amino acids that stimulate the appetite. The numbers on consumption confirm its popularity. In Italy alone, each person consumes over 23 kg per year. Yet, pasta is also extremely popular in the United States. According to the National Pasta Association, the average person in the U.S. eats 9 kg of pasta every year.

However, a 2017 study noted a decline in pasta's popularity, partly due to health and nutrition concerns. So, let's try to address some doubts.

Eating Pasta Every Day: What Happens to Our Bodies? Contrary to what some may think, eating pasta every day, as many do in Italy, is actually good for you! And most importantly, pasta does not make you gain weight. The key is to pay attention to: portion sizes, toppings, and the nutritional balance of the meal.

Here are four compelling reasons, supported by research, to enjoy it more often:

1. Energy Boost
Pasta is a food that can be enjoyed every day, provided it's consumed in moderate amounts and with nutritious toppings that improve its nutritional profile. Pasta primarily provides complex carbohydrates, essential nutrients that the body uses for energy. Its rich starch content, compared to refined sugars, takes longer to digest and provides a feeling of fullness, especially when whole grain, as it also contains soluble fibers.

2. Reduced Risk of Weight Gain

One study[1] highlighted that people who regularly eat pasta have a lower body mass index, which is associated with a lower risk of developing diseases, including cardiovascular ones. Additionally, thanks to the fiber content, regular consumption of whole grain pasta contributes to maintaining digestive health, promoting regular bowel movements.

3. What About Blood Sugar?

A 70g portion combined in the same meal with other fiber sources like vegetables and with fats and proteins, such as fish, helps to control blood sugar spikes, which over time can lead to type 2 diabetes, overweight, cardiovascular and metabolic diseases, and even cancers. Another study[2] found that pasta-based meals have a significantly lower postprandial glycemic response compared to meals based on bread or potatoes.

4. Improved Mood

The taste of a steaming plate of pasta, in addition to being a treat for the palate, also provides a boost of neurotransmitters that uplift mood. Carbohydrates in pasta, along with B-complex vitamins and tryptophan, facilitate the production of GABA, endorphins, serotonin, and melatonin. Rich in manganese and other valuable minerals that promote relaxation, pasta can even be consumed for dinner, provided that, especially if you have sleep issues, you avoid toppings rich in cheeses and sauces, which provide excessive amounts of sodium, stimulate thirst, and increase the risk of waking up in the middle of the night.

Tips for Preparing Healthy Pasta Meals:

1. Opt for whole grain, bean-based, or lentil-based pasta.
2. Add plenty of vegetables.
3. Use lean proteins, such as fish, as toppings.

1   Chiavaroli L, Kendall CWC, Braunstein CR, et alEffect of pasta in the context of low-glycaemic index dietary patterns on body weight and markers of adiposity: a systematic review and meta-analysis of randomized controlled trials in adults BMJ Open 2018;8:e019438. doi: 10.1136/bmjopen-2017-019438

2   Huang M, Li J, Ha MA, Riccardi G, Liu S. A systematic review on the relations between pasta consumption and cardio-metabolic risk factors. Nutr Metab Cardiovasc Dis. 2017 Nov;27(11):939-948. doi: 10.1016/j.numecd.2017.07.005. Epub 2017 Jul 18. PMID: 28954707.

4. Make sauces at home instead of buying pre-packaged ones.
5. Limit the amount of oil to 1-2 tablespoons.
6. Limit the portion size and aim to fill the plate with fruits and vegetables, proteins, and just over a quarter with carbohydrates.

Fruits and Vegetables

Fruits and vegetables are major players in the Mediterranean diet: their consumption of 4-5 servings per day is recommended due to their significant content of vitamins and minerals, essential micronutrients for human health. They do not provide energy but participate in numerous biological processes such as muscle contraction, bone tissue formation, red blood cell synthesis, immune system stimulation, and more. These need to be introduced through the diet because humans cannot synthesize them. It is very important to prefer fresh seasonal products of different colors. Each color in fruits and vegetables corresponds to specific substances, such as vitamins and minerals:

- **Blue-purple:** anthocyanins, carotenoids, vitamin C, potassium, and magnesium. Found in eggplants, radicchio, figs, berries, plums, black grapes.
- **Green:** vitamin C, chlorophyll, folic acid, and magnesium. Present in chicory, lettuce, arugula, zucchini, spinach, white grapes, kiwi.
- **Yellow-orange:** flavonoids, carotenoids, vitamin C. Present in oranges, lemons, grapefruits, mandarins, carrots, peppers, pumpkin, corn.
- **Red:** lycopene and anthocyanins. Present in tomatoes, radishes, watermelon, strawberries, and cherries.

Eating a colorful diet is a cornerstone principle of the Mediterranean diet, where variety is synonymous with complementarity, richness, and real balance even within the same food group.

Vegetables are also the main source of dietary fiber, which doesn't have nutritional or energetic value itself but is very important for regulating the body's various physiological functions. Dietary fiber is distinguished into:

- Water-insoluble fiber (cellulose, hemicellulose, and lignin), which primarily acts on intestinal functionality.
- Water-soluble fiber (pectins), which forms a gel upon contact with water, reducing the absorption of sugars and fats, thereby helping to control blood sugar and cholesterol levels.

Insoluble fiber is contained mainly in whole grains and vegetables, while soluble fiber is in legumes and fruit. Dietary fiber also facilitates achieving a sense of satiety, improves intestinal function, reduces the risk of chronic-degenerative diseases such as diabetes and cardiovascular diseases through the reduction of blood cholesterol levels; it's also important for the prevention of colon and rectal cancer. Although not a nutrient in the classic sense, the World Health Organization recommends an intake of about 30 grams per day.

HERE ARE THE FOODS RICHEST IN FIBER, DIVIDED BY CATEGORY:

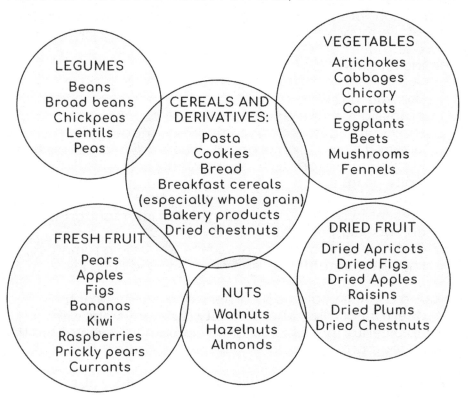

Numerous studies worldwide have shown that a diet low in fruits and vegetables doubles the risk of cancer and significantly increases the risk of heart disease and cataracts. The consumption of fruits and vegetables seems to be protective, especially against cancers of the mouth, larynx, esophagus, stomach, and intestines; it can help control weight and reduce the risk of diabetes and high blood pressure. Useful components include vitamin C and various carotenoids, including beta-carotene, which can be converted into vitamin A in the body.

These substances are also important as antioxidants that help defend against free radicals involved in aging. Vegetables also provide minerals, particularly iron, calcium, magnesium, potassium, and dietary fiber. Depending on the type, fiber helps regulate intestinal functions and control blood sugar and cholesterol levels.

Finally, fruits and vegetables also provide a large amount of biologically-active compounds, called "phytochemicals," thought to promote health and reduce the risk of diseases. Among these are indoles from broccoli, cabbages, and other cruciferous vegetables; isoflavones from soybeans; allile sulfur compounds from garlic and onions, phenolic acids from tomatoes and carrots, and many others. The artichoke, a typical Mediterranean vegetable, is undoubtedly a source of antioxidants and other important active principles.

In conclusion, the protective effect of vegetables is likely due not to a single component but to a wide variety of substances, partly known and partly yet to be discovered, that act in association with each other.

Vegetable Functionality

The **liliaceae** family (garlic, onion, leek, shallot, chives, etc.) has been used for millennia for its medicinal properties. Those colored yellow or red are excellent sources of quercetin. More generally, they may have the following properties: antibacterial, antitumor, stroke risk reduction, inhibition of nitrosamine formation (teratogens).

Garlic contains substances that can prevent hypertension and high cholesterol. However, recent trials have found that the intake of garlic oil capsules (extracted via steam distillation) has no significant effect on cholesterol synthesis and absorption. Garlic has antibacterial efficacy; added to preparations of only partially cooked meat, it reduces the microbial load of Escherichia coli, a bacterium capable of inducing severe gastrointestinal disorders, by 75%. Its consumption reduces the risk of stomach cancer. Much of garlic's protective qualities are attributed to the sulfur compounds (with the classic pungent smell) contained in its husk.

Onions contain flavonoids (powerful antioxidants) and sulfur compounds useful in the prevention of cancer and cardiovascular diseases (they reduce platelet aggregation, decreasing the risk of thrombus formation). They have a diuretic and disinfectant action.

Cruciferous vegetables (cabbages, cauliflowers, broccoli, etc.) contain substances, such as glucosinolates (sulfur compounds), that reduce cancer risk, particularly referring to colorectal cancer.

Broccoli and cabbages contain several phytochemical substances that protect against cancer: such as sulforaphane, which boosts enzymes that detoxify cells, and isothiocyanate, which neutralizes carcinogens and prevents DNA damage.

Chicory is a good source of calcium, iron, potassium, carotenoids, vitamin E, and fiber. Its roots contain inulin, a specific fiber that promotes the growth of bifidobacteria in the intestinal flora (known for its probiotic effect).

Spinach is among the most nutrient-rich vegetables, containing high amounts of vitamins C and E, beta-carotene, as well as lutein and zeaxanthin, which seem to prevent aging and degeneration of the eye's macula. They also contain good amounts of potassium, folic acid, dietary fiber, and iron (which, however, is in a form not readily available). The high content of oxalic acid makes them unsuitable for those suffering from oxalic kidney stones.

Umbelliferae (carrots, celery, parsley) contain several phytochemical substances in their oil fraction that boost the detoxifying and anticancer action of the enzyme Glutathione-S-transferase.
Carrots are an excellent source of beta-carotene (60 grams of carrots provide a quantity equivalent to the recommended daily level of vitamin A), as well as potassium and fiber. Recently, the contribution of other antioxidants, such as lycopene and canthaxanthin, has been valued.

Apples are a good source of vitamin B (biotin), minerals, soluble fiber. They contain polyphenolic antioxidants in the skin and pulp.
Peaches are a good source of vitamin B3 (niacin). Yellow-fleshed ones are a significant source of carotenoids. Contains phytosterols (plant estrogens) and glutathione.

Apricots are a good source of carotenoids and potassium. Plums are a good source of vitamins C and B2 (riboflavin). They have excellent antioxidant capacity, which does not diminish with dehydration. Dried plums, in fact, have a very high antioxidant capacity, as well as a good content of calcium.

Cherries and sour cherries are a good source of vitamin C, and sour cherries, in particular, of carotenoids. Darker-colored ones contain significant amounts of anthocyanins.

Oranges and lemons, besides being an excellent source of vitamin C, contain other substances with anticancer activity: monoterpenes (mostly d-limonene), glutathione, folic acid, and, in the case of blood oranges, anthocyanins. The d-limonene is contained in the peel. It has not been verified if the anticancer activity persists in jams.

Grapes are a good source of vitamin C and, especially in the case of red grapes, phenolic compounds with high antioxidant power (such as resveratrol), which are also found in red wine. It also contains caffeic acid.

Berries, blackberries, and strawberries are among the vegetables with the highest antioxidant capacity measured in laboratory tests, as well as the ability to reverse some effects of aging: loss of balance, coordination, and memory.
Their high antioxidant power has been attributed in part to the content of vitamin C and mostly to the content of phenolic substances. Blackberries are also a good source of saponins, substances that can reduce plasma cholesterol levels. Blueberries contain an undefined factor that prevents bacteria from adhering to the bladder wall, preventing infections.

Figs are an excellent source of calcium and polyphenols, which are concentrated in dried figs. Their extracts have shown significant antibacterial activity and a potential antitumoral effect. In addition to polyphenols, they also contain benzaldehyde and coumarins, a class of substances with anticoagulant effects tested in the treatment of prostate and skin cancer.

The Tomato

The tomato, a cornerstone of the Mediterranean diet, is celebrated for its numerous health benefits, derived from a rich nutritional composition. This vegetable stands out for its culinary versatility and the broad spectrum of nutrients it offers. Among these, potassium, phosphorus, folates, and vitamin C—the latter mainly present in its raw version due to its sensitivity to heat. With a calorie content of only 18 calories per 100 grams, the tomato fits perfectly into low-calorie diets as well, thanks to its low caloric content and high water percentage.

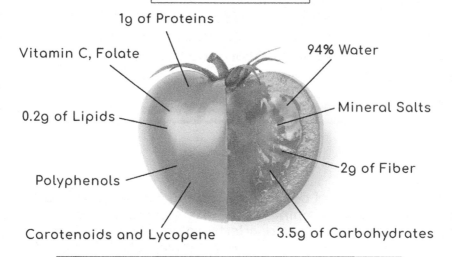

THE TOMATO

1g of Proteins

Vitamin C, Folate

94% Water

0.2g of Lipids

Mineral Salts

Polyphenols

2g of Fiber

Carotenoids and Lycopene

3.5g of Carbohydrates

Simplified diagram of some of the
main characteristic constituents of the tomato.

The added value of the tomato lies in its abundance of antioxidants, such as lycopene, which not only gives it its characteristic red color but also plays a crucial role in cellular protection against the action of free radicals, thereby delaying aging and reducing the risk of degenerative and cardiovascular diseases. Lycopene, along with other antioxidants present such as polyphenols and carotenoids, contributes to a range of positive health effects.

Among the main benefits of the tomato are its anti-aging action, the boosting of the immune system, the promotion of digestion thanks to its organic acids and fibers, the diuretic effect due to its high potassium content, which combats water retention, and the support to visual health, particularly through the antioxidant zeaxanthin which protects against cataracts and macular degeneration.

Despite these virtues, tomatoes may not be suitable for everyone. Some individuals might experience allergic reactions due to the proteins and histamine they contain, or aggravate conditions such as heartburn, reflux, gastritis, or ulcers due to the acids and lectin present.

Moreover, the solanine found in the skin of unripe tomatoes can cause gastrointestinal disturbances. Therefore, while being an excellent health ally for many, its consumption should be carefully evaluated in the presence of specific medical conditions.

Legumes, Fish, Eggs, and Meat

Proteins are crucial components of our body and contain so-called essential amino acids, which the body processes from foods. Proteins are divided into animal (meat, fish, eggs, cheese, poultry, milk) and plant (cereals, legumes, nuts). Animal proteins are considered more valuable, while plant proteins have a lower biological value but present the effect of "complementation," which consists of enhancing their biological value when appropriately paired. Cereals, combined with legumes, have a biological value similar to that of meat, which is why it's possible to live healthily on a strictly vegetarian diet.

The Mediterranean diet favors plant proteins paired with carbohydrates, milk derivatives, and eggs, and also suggests a weekly consumption of fish and white meats while indicating red meats should be consumed only a few times a month. Diets high in animal proteins, especially red meat, can promote cancer, particularly liver, colorectal, kidney, and breast cancer.

Literature data suggest that consuming fish once or more a week is associated with a reduction in the incidence of ischemic heart disease. The effect of reducing cardiovascular risk factors for the intake of significant doses of omega-3 is also manifested compared to a vegetarian diet, which itself seems to have a similar protective function.

Oily fish (mackerel and sardines) and salmon are good sources of omega-3 (over 2 grams per average serving), even when preserved by canning or smoking. Omega-3 fatty acids are polyunsaturated fatty acids and can be considered "essential" as they are not synthesized in our bodies, despite playing very important biological functions. Mainly contained in fish oil, they reduce the risk of cardiovascular diseases and act on the nervous system with an antidepressant effect.

Finally, meats and fish are also important sources of bioavailable iron. Significant amounts of iron are also contained in plant foods, but its absorption is much more limited if not combined with the simultaneous intake of vitamin C sources. Iron is essential for health and the proper functioning of hemoglobin, responsible for transporting oxygen to all body cells. The first symptoms of iron deficiency are fatigue and exhaustion, worsening of memory and learning capacity.

Milk and Byproducts

Due to their high calcium content, they are particularly recommended in the diet of children, women, and the elderly, to ensure good growth and maintenance of bones. Mediterranean dietary regimes recommend consuming 1-2 servings of milk and byproducts per day, preferring those with low fat content.
While low-fat yogurt can be consumed every day, it's better not to consume aged cheeses more than 4-5 times a week because they also contain high concentrations of fats.
The suggestion is to opt for less processed dairy: consider flavorful cheeses like Parmesan, feta, or partially skimmed mozzarella instead of highly processed American cheese slices. Speaking of yogurt, plain Greek yogurt is the best, while flavored varieties high in sugar should be avoided.

Fermented Foods

Ilya Ilyich Mechnikov, a Russian biologist and immunologist who won the Nobel Prize in Medicine, conducted innovative studies on longevity, correlating it with the intake of fermented milk. This food, along with other fermented products like yogurt, sourdough bread, cheese, wine, beer, sauerkraut, and cured meats, has a long history in human nutrition, especially in Mediterranean cultures, thanks to their durability, safety, and organoleptic properties.

Recent research has highlighted that fermented foods can offer health benefits thanks to fermenting microorganisms and the bioactive products resulting from fermentation. Some of these microorganisms are similar to probiotic strains, suggesting that regular consumption of fermented foods can have very positive effects on health.

In particular, dairy products derived from fermented milk like yogurt have been shown to positively influence human health, associated with maintaining body weight, reducing the risk of cardiovascular diseases, type 2 diabetes, and improving glucose metabolism. Other studies have shown benefits for inflammatory bowel diseases and brain health, suggesting that fermented foods can positively influence mood and brain activity through the microbiota-gut-brain axis.

A Mediterranean diet enriched with fermented dairy products can significantly improve cardiovascular risk factors. For all these reasons, research continues to explore how fermented foods of all kinds, integrated into a Mediterranean diet, can contribute to a longer and healthier life.

Seasonings and Olive Oil

Culturally, we're accustomed to seeing seasonings and fats as something to avoid and watch out for, but in the Mediterranean diet, olive oil is a fundamental ingredient that is not only not feared but is highly recommended.

This is because not all fats are equal, and not all are harmful. We can fundamentally distinguish fats into saturated and unsaturated; the former contribute to raising the cholesterol content in the blood, the latter lower it. Animal fats (butter, bacon, lard, suet) belong to the first category, while vegetable fats (nuts, seed oil, extra virgin olive oil) belong to the second.

Extra virgin olive oil is particularly rich in monounsaturated fats and oleic acid and is among the best allies for controlling the level of "bad" cholesterol. Its consumption should only be moderated if following a weight loss diet because, although rich in very useful principles, it retains a high caloric value. Other "good" unsaturated fats, omega-3 fatty acids present in plant-based foods like various seeds and nuts, as well as in fatty fish like anchovies, salmon, herring, mackerels, play an important role in preventing cardiovascular and cancerous diseases.

Seeds and nuts like walnuts, almonds, hazelnuts, and chestnuts are particularly rich in antioxidants. Until a few years ago, nuts were on the blacklist of nutrition, and even doctors advised against their consumption, but now we know that nearly daily consumption of them can help halve the risk of heart diseases. The effect is attributed to their "good" fatty fraction composed of monounsaturated fatty acids and vitamin E, which also has the ability to improve the lipid profile in the blood and increase its resistance to oxidation, thus preventing atherosclerosis.

Among the seasonings, it's worth noting that the Mediterranean diet includes extensive use of garlic, aromatic herbs, and many spices: sage, cinnamon, and oregano not only add aroma and flavor to dishes but limit the proliferation of bacteria and have a high antioxidant power.

Extra Virgin Olive Oil

EVOO (Extra Virgin Olive Oil) has all the optimal characteristics to be considered the basis of the Mediterranean diet. In the Mediterranean diet, only extra virgin is considered because, being made from selected, healthy olives and cold-pressed, it manages to retain all the therapeutic characteristics and main nutrients, which are: unsaturated fatty acids, especially oleic acid, polyphenols, and vitamin A. Scientific studies demonstrate that this food manages to maintain our body's wellbeing and prevent chronic metabolic diseases. The use of olive oil is very varied and applicable to different types of cooking and culinary preparation:

- **Raw** extra virgin olive oil enhances the aroma and flavor of the food it dresses: salads, sauces, dipping, bread, toast, sandwiches, preserved in oil, etc. A universe of combinations where the quality of the extra virgin makes all the difference.

- For **sautéing, pan-frying, and stewing:** the cooking happens with the steam released by the food, like meat, fish, legumes, and vegetables, EVOO creates an outer layer that intensifies the flavors of the dishes even more and allows to maintain the therapeutic properties of the foods making the result healthier and tastier.

- **Baking:** normally, meats or fish baked in the oven deteriorate and dry out too much if fats are not added. Extra virgin olive oil, being rich in oleic acid, withstands high temperatures well, and the result is juicier and healthier since it protects the food.

- **Grilling:** EVOO helps to cook the food and makes a film that prevents the food from sticking to the grill. When grilling, EVOO is added after cooking to soften the dry parts due to contact with the charcoal.

- **Frying:** virgin olive oil is the most stable of vegetable fats and does not produce toxic reactions when fried, roasted, or cooked, under normal conditions, as long as the temperature is kept below 356°F. On the contrary, it improves the gastronomic qualities of food. During frying, it forms a thin and consistent layer around the product, which prevents it from absorbing more oil and allows it to retain all the flavors. Olive oil fries and does not cook, unlike most other oils.

It's time to dispel the myth that EVOO is only for raw dressings. It's essential to understand that extra virgin olive oil is a valid fat for any culinary application and, besides the benefits of the oil itself, allows all the properties of the foods to be preserved and makes every dish more digestible. Furthermore, if the EVOO we choose is organic, we have more guarantees that, in addition to eating well, we are also eating healthily.

Water and Other Beverages

Beyond food, there's another element, at the base of the "food pyramid," that can contribute to safeguarding heart health and can prove to be an excellent weapon for defense against cardiovascular problems: water.

A well-hydrated body can reduce the viscosity of the blood and the consequent risk of thrombosis within the blood vessels, and even regulate blood pressure, especially for those suffering from hypertension. Water's importance for the heart also comes from the minerals it can contain, with magnesium and calcium being two essential elements to prevent the risk of numerous cardiovascular complications, as they can influence the contraction capacity of cardiovascular muscles and reduce blood fats. Magnesium promotes the relaxation of cardiac muscle fibrocells, while calcium stimulates the contraction of cardiac muscle cells, intervening in the blood thinning and thus reducing heart attack risks. It's recommended to drink 1.5 to 2 liters per day (about six to eight glasses).

Besides water, coffee, tea, and herbal infusions (rich in flavonoids) can also be consumed, but it's better without sugar or with half a teaspoon of honey, avoiding the use of sweeteners.

Wine is also present in the Mediterranean diet pyramid, provided religious and social beliefs allow it, with moderate consumption recommended: one glass per day for women and two for men. It has been shown that modest alcohol consumption has beneficial effects on cardiovascular diseases as it increases good cholesterol are attributed to resveratrol, a natural antioxidant mainly contained in red wines. Other beneficial compounds include procyanidins and proanthocyanidins, which improve the elasticity of blood vessels.

Summary Table

Many foods and ingredients of the Mediterranean diet are also widely used in the United States, simple foods that can commonly be found in supermarkets and are probably at the base of your favorite dishes. The choice is vast:

VEGETABLES & TUBERS ▲▲▲

artichokes, arugula, beets, broccoli, brussels sprouts, cabbage, carrots, celery, celeriac, chicory, collard cucumber, dandelion greens, eggplant, fennel, kale, leeks, lettuce, mâche, mushrooms, mustard greens, nettles, okra, onions (red, sweet, white), peas, peppers, potatoes, purslane, radishes, rutabaga, scallions,

GRAINS ▲▲▲

breads, barley, buckwheat, bulgur, couscous, durum, farro, freekeh, millet, oats, polenta, rice, wheat berries

POULTRY & EGGS ▲▲

chicken, duck, guinea fowl, quail chicken eggs, duck eggs, quail eggs

FRUITS ▲▲▲

avocados, apples, apricots, cherries, clementines, dates, figs, grapefruit, grapes, lemons, melons, nectarines, olives, oranges, peaches, pears, pomegranates, pumpkin, strawberries, tangerines, tomatoes

FISH & SEAFOOD ▲▲

abalone, cockles, clams, crab, eel, flounder, lobster, mackerel, mussels, octopus, oysters, salmon, sardines, sea bass, shrimp, squid, tilapia, tuna, whelk, yellowtail

SWEETS ▲

treats made with fruits, nuts, whole grains, and minimal sugars

baklava, biscotti, crème caramel, chocolate, gelato, kunefe, lokum (Turkish delight), mousse au chocolat, sorbet

NUTS, SEEDS, & LEGUMES ▲▲▲

almonds, beans (cannellini, chickpeas, fava, green, kidney), cashews, hazelnuts, lentils, pine nuts, pistachios, sesame seeds (tahini), split peas, walnuts

HERBS & SPICES ▲▲▲

anise, basil, bay leaf, chiles, clove, cumin, fennel, garlic, lavender, marjoram, mint, oregano, parsley, pepper, pul biber (Aleppo pepper), rosemary, sage, savory, sumac, tarragon, thyme, za'atar

CHEESE & YOGURT ▲▲

Brie, Chevre, Corvo, feta, Halloumi, Manchego, Parmigiano-Reggiano, Pecorino, ricotta Greek yogurt

MEATS ▲

beef, goat, lamb, mutton, pork

▲▲▲ EAT MOST OFTEN
▲▲ EAT MODERATELY
▲ EAT LESS OFTEN

Mediterranean Eating for Beginners

The Mediterranean diet pyramid and the "Healthy Eating Plate" provide a general model on food groups to include in every meal. However, especially when starting a dietary plan, many doubts may arise. To avoid mistakes, the advice is to fill your plate in this way:

- half fruits and vegetables,
- a quarter whole grains,
- and a quarter healthy proteins.

The Mediterranean diet is intentionally vague about specific foods, making the diet adaptable to individual preferences and applicable to various types of cuisine and taste preferences, such as those following a plant-based diet. In the Mediterranean diet, there are no real "forbidden" foods, but there are those whose consumption should be very moderate. Alternating ingredients, favoring variety and seasonality, rather than always eating the same things, has a further double advantage: not getting bored, being able to maintain the diet in the long term, and offering the body a wide range of different nutrients.

Here are some recommendations to start simply:

- Vegetables
Their colors should always be the stars of the plate. Fruits and vegetables should make up the majority of your meals. Think of small ways to add more vegetables to your meals, such as adding spinach to your eggs, loading your sandwich with avocado and tomato, making an eggplant sauce, or using a piece of fruit as a snack. If you eat yogurt for breakfast, add chopped fruit or berries. Dried or dried fruit is also a tasty way to reach the recommended daily doses.

- Choose Natural Foods
Whenever possible, only put raw materials in your cart instead of prepared products. This means choosing ingredients like legumes or whole grains such as oats and bulgur, fruits, vegetables, fish, and healthy vegetable oils like olive oil. The better the quality of the raw materials: the healthier and more nutritious your meal will be.

- Opt for Whole Grains
Being among the most present foods, choosing whole grains instead of refined ones really makes a big difference. Whole grain products have the ability to lower cholesterol, balance blood glucose levels, and facilitate body weight management; they are rich in B vitamins and fibers, contributing to general well-being.

- Eat Nuts
Nuts, like vegetable oils and avocado, contain poly- and monounsaturated fats beneficial for cardiovascular health. They are also a source of proteins and fibers, help maintain satiety, stabilize blood sugar levels, reduce cholesterol, and fight inflammation. The simplest way to remember to eat them is to include them in breakfast or use them as snacks to avoid arriving at meals too hungry.

- The Advantages of Fish
Fatty fish such as salmon, mackerel, tuna, and herring are the main sources of protein in the Mediterranean diet. These fish contain high doses of omega-3 fatty acids, which help reduce inflammation and improve cholesterol levels. Additionally, if you don't have access to fresh fish, canned versions of these are just as nutritious, quicker to prepare, and last much longer in your pantry. White fish and seafood are also good sources of lean protein but are not as rich in omega-3.

- Replace Butter with Olive Oil
Healthy vegetable oils like olive oil are a main source of fats in the Mediterranean diet, and the quality of the type of fat is more important than the quantity. The goal is to consume only heart-healthy fats (poly- and monounsaturated fats) and always less saturated and trans fats. The best vegetable oils are olive, canola, avocado, and peanut oil.

- Reconsider Dairy
In moderation, try to eat a variety of tasty cheeses or dairy products and avoid the saturated fats of cream. In the Mediterranean diet, the most common cheeses are feta or Parmesan, while American cheese is unfortunately one of the most processed.
Natural yogurt, low-fat yogurt, and Greek yogurt are permitted and advisable even daily, avoid those high in sugar by reading labels carefully.

- Limit Added Sugars

Sweets might be one of the major sacrifices; the Mediterranean diet almost completely avoids the consumption of refined sugars, limiting them to special occasions or just a couple of servings a week. For daily cravings, prefer natural fruit, which satisfies the need for sweetness while providing useful nutrients. Again, it's a matter of habit... It's known that sugars create a strong addiction, so at first, it might be difficult, but over time it will become normal, and the health benefits will be enormous.

7 Easy Mediterranean Swaps

Gradual and gentle changes in one's life always have a better chance of taking root and lasting over time. That's why one of the simplest ways to adhere to the Mediterranean diet is to start with six easy food swaps that help you eat healthier without overhauling your life. There's no need to radically change everything at once, but to start, you can make some small changes based on the simple principles of the Mediterranean way of eating every day. This will immediately transform your favorite dishes into healthier, nutrient-rich, and delicious options.

1. Swap butter and processed oils for extra virgin olive oil. Butter is high in saturated fats and can contribute to high cholesterol levels, while extra virgin olive oil is loaded with healthy monounsaturated fats and polyphenols that promote heart health and reduce inflammation.

2. Replace red meat with fish or lean and plant-based proteins. Instead of relying on meat such as steaks or sausages for protein, try healthier and more affordable options like chicken, fish, or legumes.

3. Incorporate whole grains instead of refined ones into your diet. When shopping, choose whole grain bread, pasta, and flours instead of their white counterparts.

4. Cut back or eliminate sugary drinks in favor of water or herbal tea is another step towards a healthier diet. Sugary drinks are full of empty calories and added sugars, which in the food pyramid are placed right at the top among the foods to drastically reduce.

5. If you're craving a snack, prefer fresh and natural snacks over processed ones such as fresh fruit, vegetable sticks, hummus, or a handful of raw nuts that offer vitamins, minerals, and healthy fats. It's just a matter of habit!

6. Choose low-fat dairy products like feta, ricotta, and lean cheeses. You can replace mayonnaise with yogurt or yogurt-based sauces.

7. Opt for spices instead of salt; this small change can reduce sodium intake and add flavor to dishes with health benefits.

Small changes can lead to big results. Starting today takes you one step forward towards a healthier and happier life.

Mediterranean Pantry List

FRUITS & VEGETABLES

Select an assortment of hues and opt for seasonal produce to maximize nutritional benefits. Frozen and canned varieties are also excellent choices for affordability and extended shelf life — just ensure they contain little to no added salt, sugar, or fats.

Apples	Brussels sprouts
Apricots	Cabbage
Avocado	Collards (from
Bananas	Greens section)
Berries	Greens (includes
Cherries	kale, spinach,
Clementines	collards, arugula)
Dates	Onions
Figs	Peas
Grapes	Peppers
Oranges	Potatoes
Pears	Spinach (from
Artichokes	Greens section)
Arugula	Tomatoes
Beets	Zucchini

POULTRY

These lean meats are acceptable within the Mediterranean diet, but should be consumed less frequently.

Chicken
Turkey

MEAT

Eat these protein-rich meats intermittently, too. Combine a small portion with whole grains and vegetables for a balanced meal.

Pork
Beef
Lamb (a few times per month or less)

HERBS & SPICES

Rather than depending on the salt shaker, purchase a selection of these to enhance your meals. Fresh herbs are tasty, but dried ones are effective as well; just reduce the quantity used to achieve a comparable taste, as they tend to be more concentrated.

Parsley	Dill
Cilantro	Sage
Ginger	Rosemary
Garlic	Tarragon
Mint	Basil
Thyme	Oregano

WHOLE GRAINS

Combine different options to create fast and effortless side dishes, the foundation for grain bowls, or straightforward grain-based stir-fries.

Whole-grain breads	Buckwheat
Corn	Farro
Oats	Barley
Brown rice	Couscous
Bulgur	Wheat berries

FISH

Strive to consume more fish compared to other sources of animal protein. Canned and frozen varieties provide excellent alternatives that have a longer shelf life than fresh options, yet still deliver equivalent nutritional advantages.

Salmon
Tuna
Mackerel
Herring and sardines
Other seafood as desired

DAIRY

Dairy is permitted in the Mediterranean diet, but should be consumed in moderation.

Feta	Ricotta
Brie	Manchego
Cotija	Parmesan
Swiss	Plain yogurt
Halloumi	Greek yogurt

NUTS, SEEDS & LEGUMES

Select a variety as preferred for snacks, toppings for salads, and additional uses.

Chickpeas	Walnuts
Black beans	Almonds
Kidney beans	Hazelnuts
Pinto beans	Cashews
Lentils (all types)	Pine nuts
Fava beans	Sesame seeds

OTHER MEDITERRANEAN DIET STAPLES

Olive oil
Canola oil
Avocado oil
Seanut oil
Sesame oil
Eggs
Red wine

MEDITERRANEAN RECIPES

Starting to eat Mediterranean doesn't mean making drastic changes, but rather gradual substitutions and acquiring the ability to compose balanced dishes where the focus is always on good portions of vegetables, a part of whole grains, and a smaller part of proteins, obviously good ones.
The recipes you find in this section of the book are simple, mostly very quick, with which you can start to familiarize yourself and become comfortable in the kitchen with the new dietary style.
You will find all these dishes within the four-week Meal Plan.

Always remember that the Mediterranean diet is a flexible diet, what counts are:

- proportions on the plate
- variety of ingredients
- portion sizes (especially if you need to lose weight)
- seasonality of products.

Feel free to modify these recipes according to your taste or what you find available in supermarkets. When you choose to make a substitution, stay true to the quantities and the food group within which you are applying the substitution. For example, you can replace tuna with salmon, chicken with turkey, use spinach instead of broccoli, etc... If you have doubts, you can use the table from the previous pages.

Dietary Tags:

V: Vegetarian, without meat, fish. May include dairy products and eggs.

VG: Vegan, completely free of animal products, including dairy, eggs, and honey.

EF: Egg-Free. Recipes that do not contain eggs.

DF: Dairy-Free. Recipes without milk and milk-derived products.

HF: High-Fiber.

GF: Gluten-Free. Suitable for those with celiac disease or gluten sensitivity.

NF: Nut-Free. Recipes that do not contain nuts or nut-derived products.

BREAKFAST RECIPES

Orange-Spiced Overnight Oats | V, EF, DF, HF, GF

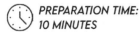 *PREPARATION TIME:*
10 MINUTES

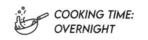 *COOKING TIME:*
OVERNIGHT

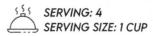 *SERVING: 4*
SERVING SIZE: 1 CUP

Ingredients

- 1 3/4 cups cashew milk, plus more for serving
- 1 tbsp honey, warmed, plus more for drizzling if desired
- 2 tsp orange zest plus 3/4 cup orange juice
- 3/4 tsp ground cinnamon
- 1/4 tsp kosher salt
- 1 1/2 cups rolled oats
- 2 tbsp chia seeds
- 3 oranges, peeled and cut into segments
- 2/3 cup chopped almonds
- Walnut kernels, for serving

Directions

1. In a large bowl, combine cashew milk, warmed honey, orange zest and juice, cinnamon, and salt.
2. Stir in the oats and chia seeds. Cover and refrigerate overnight.
3. If desired, alter the consistency by adding more cashew milk. Roughly chop half of the orange segments and fold them into the grains with half of the almonds.
4. Top each serving with the remaining whole orange segments, the rest of the chopped almonds, additional honey, and walnut kernels.

Nutrition information per serving
Calories: 365; Protein: 9g; Carbs: 47g; Fiber: 9g; Fat: 18g

Peach and Raspberry Greek Yogurt Bowl | V, GF, NF

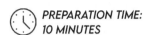 **PREPARATION TIME:**
10 MINUTES

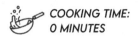 **COOKING TIME:**
0 MINUTES

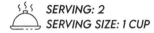 **SERVING: 2**
SERVING SIZE: 1 CUP

Ingredients

- 1 cup fresh peaches, sliced
- 1 cup fresh raspberries
- 2 cups non-fat plain Greek yogurt
- 1/4 cup unsweetened almond milk
- 1 tbsp chia seeds
- 1 tbsp ground flaxseed
- 1 tsp cinnamon

Directions

1. In a medium bowl, mix together the non-fat plain Greek yogurt and unsweetened almond milk.
2. Stir in the chia seeds, ground flaxseed, and cinnamon. Allow the mixture to sit for about 5 minutes to thicken.
3. Evenly distribute the yogurt mixture into two bowls.
4. Garnish each bowl with sliced peaches and fresh raspberries. Serve immediately.

Nutrition information per serving
Calories: 220; Carbs: 27g; Fat: 5g; Protein: 17g; Fiber: 9g

Seasonal Fruit Breakfast Bowl | VG, EF, DF, HF, GF

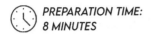 **PREPARATION TIME:**
8 MINUTES

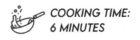 **COOKING TIME:**
6 MINUTES

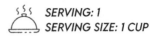 **SERVING: 1**
SERVING SIZE: 1 CUP

Ingredients

- 1 cup unsweetened almond milk
- 1 cup whole-grain oats
- 1/2 cup apricot chunks (or peaches, pineapple, mango, or any other seasonal fruit)
- 2 tablespoons chopped walnuts
- 1 tablespoon unsweetened coconut flakes

Directions

1. Combine the almond milk and oats in a small, microwave-safe bowl.
2. Microwave on high for 6 minutes.
3. Stir, then let it stand for 2 minutes.
4. Top with apricot chunks (or your choice of seasonal fruit), walnuts, and coconut flakes.

Nutrition information per serving

Calories: 333; Fat: 18.1g; Carbs: 38g; Protein: 8.2g; Fiber: 8g;

Quinoa Porridge with Banana and Walnuts
VG, EF, DF, GF

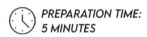 **PREPARATION TIME:** 5 MINUTES

 **COOKING TIME:** 20 MINUTES

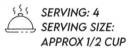 **SERVING: 4** SERVING SIZE: APPROX 1/2 CUP

Ingredients

- 1 cup quinoa, rinsed and drained
- 2 cups unsweetened almond milk
- 1/2 tsp ground cinnamon
- Pinch of sea salt
- 2 ripe bananas, thinly sliced
- 1/4 cup chopped walnuts

Directions

1. In a medium saucepan, combine quinoa, almond milk, cinnamon, and a pinch of sea salt. Place over medium heat and bring to a boil.
2. Once boiling, reduce heat to low and let the quinoa simmer for 20 minutes, or until fully cooked, stirring occasionally to prevent sticking.
3. Remove from heat. Gently fold in the sliced bananas and chopped walnuts until evenly distributed throughout the porridge.
4. Serve the quinoa porridge warm, divided into bowls.

Nutrition information per serving
Calories: 275; Carbs: 37g; Fat: 10g; Protein: 9g; Fiber: 6g

Chia Pudding with Fresh Fruit | V, EF, GF, NF

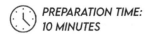 **PREPARATION TIME:** 10 MINUTES

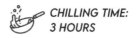 **CHILLING TIME:** 3 HOURS

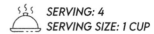 **SERVING: 4** SERVING SIZE: 1 CUP

Ingredients

- 1/4 cup chia seeds
- 1 cup unsweetened almond milk
- 1/2 cup non-fat Greek yogurt
- 1 tbsp honey (optional)
- 1 tsp vanilla extract
- 1 cup mixed fresh fruit (e.g., berries, mango, kiwi)
- Fresh mint leaves for garnishing (optional)

Directions

1. In a medium bowl, whisk together chia seeds, unsweetened almond milk, non-fat Greek yogurt, honey (if using), and vanilla extract. Ensure all ingredients are well combined.
2. Cover the bowl with a lid or plastic wrap and refrigerate for at least 3 hours, allowing the chia seeds to swell and the pudding to thicken.
3. Once the pudding has set, stir well. Divide the chia pudding evenly among four serving glasses or bowls.
4. Top each serving with a generous portion of mixed fresh fruit. If desired, garnish with fresh mint leaves for an added touch of freshness.

Nutrition information per serving

Calories: 134; Carbs: 16g; Fat: 5g; Protein: 7g; Fiber: 7g

Yogurt with Bananas and Almond-Buckwheat Groats

V, EF, HF, GF

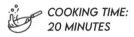 **PREPARATION TIME:** 20 MINUTES   **COOKING TIME:** 20 MINUTES   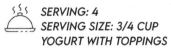 **SERVING: 4** **SERVING SIZE: 3/4 CUP YOGURT WITH TOPPINGS**

Ingredients

- 1 tbsp. olive oil
- 1 1/2 tbsp. pure maple syrup, divided
- Kosher salt
- 1/2 cup buckwheat groats
- 1/4 tsp. chia seeds
- 1/3 cup sliced almonds
- 1 lb. bananas, thickly sliced
- 3 cups Greek yogurt

Directions

1. Preheat the oven to 300°F. Line a small rimmed baking sheet with parchment paper. In a bowl, whisk together olive oil, 1 tablespoon maple syrup, and 1/4 teaspoon salt.
2. Heat a medium cast-iron skillet on medium-high. Add groats and toast, shaking and tossing often and adjusting heat as needed, until color and aroma deepen and groats are crisp, 1 to 2 minutes.
3. Transfer toasted groats to the bowl with maple syrup mixture and toss to coat. Stir in chia seeds and almonds. Spread onto the prepared baking sheet and bake, stirring halfway through and rotating the baking sheet, until golden brown, about 15 to 20 minutes. Let cool.
4. In a bowl, toss bananas with the remaining 1/2 tablespoon maple syrup and a pinch of salt; let sit for 5 minutes.
5. To serve, spoon bananas and juices over Greek yogurt; top with almond-buckwheat groats. Store leftover groats in an airtight container at room temperature for up to 10 days.

Nutrition information per serving

Calories: 332; Protein: 20g; Fat: 17g; Carbs: 27g; Fiber: 4g;

Greek Yogurt Berry Parfait | V, EF, GF

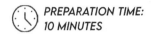 **PREPARATION TIME:** 10 MINUTES   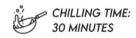 **CHILLING TIME:** 30 MINUTES   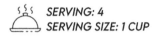 **SERVING: 4** SERVING SIZE: 1 CUP

Ingredients

- 2 cups low-fat Greek yogurt
- 1 cup mixed berries (blueberries, raspberries, and strawberries)
- 1/4 cup unsweetened almond milk
- 1 tbsp honey
- 1 tsp vanilla extract
- 8 tbsp chia seeds
- Optional: fresh mint leaves for garnish

Directions

1. In a medium bowl, mix the low-fat Greek yogurt with unsweetened almond milk and honey. Stir in the vanilla extract.
2. Begin to assemble the parfaits by placing a layer of the Greek yogurt mixture into four individual serving cups.
3. Add a layer of mixed berries on top of the yogurt in each cup, then sprinkle chia seeds over the berries.
4. Repeat the layers with the remaining Greek yogurt mixture and mixed berries, finishing with a final sprinkle of chia seeds on top.
5. Refrigerate the parfaits for at least 30 minutes to allow the chia seeds to hydrate and expand.
6. Optional: Garnish with fresh mint leaves before serving.

Nutrition information per serving
Calories: 160; Carbs: 13g; Fat: 6g; Protein: 12g; Fiber: 5g

Strawberries Banana Smoothie Delight | V, EF, GF

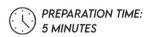 **PREPARATION TIME:** 5 MINUTES
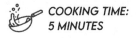 **COOKING TIME:** 5 MINUTES
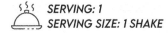 **SERVING: 1** SERVING SIZE: 1 SHAKE

Ingredients

- 1/2 cup strawberries
- 1/2 ripe frozen banana
- 1/2 cup organic nonfat frozen yogurt
- 1/2 cup unsweetened vanilla almond milk (or skim, soy, etc.)

Directions

1. Place all ingredients in a blender.
2. Blend until smooth.

Nutrition information per serving
Calories: 211; Carbs: 48g; Fat: 2.1g; Protein: 5.6g; Fiber: 5.7g

Tropical Fruit Yogurt Delight | V, EF, GF, HF

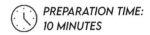 **PREPARATION TIME:**
10 MINUTES

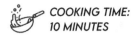 **COOKING TIME:**
10 MINUTES

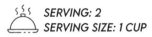 **SERVING: 2**
SERVING SIZE: 1 CUP

Ingredients

- 1 cup tropical fruit, diced (e.g., mango, pineapple, papaya)
- 1 1/2 tablespoons raw sugar
- 1 tablespoon golden raisins
- 1/4 cup desiccated coconut
- A pinch of nutmeg
- 2 cups 0% fat plain Greek yogurt
- 4 tablespoons chopped walnuts or pecans

Directions

1. In a small pot, combine the diced tropical fruit, raw sugar, and golden raisins. Add 1/4 cup water, sprinkle with nutmeg. Cover and cook over low heat until the fruit is soft, about 6 to 7 minutes. Set aside to cool.
2. Divide the Greek yogurt between two medium bowls.
3. Top each bowl with the tropical fruit mixture and sprinkle with desiccated coconut and chopped nuts. Serve immediately.

Nutrition information per serving
Calories: 283; Carbs: 40g; Fat: 10g; Protein: 12.5g; Fiber: 3g

Almond Flour Berry Pancakes | V, DF, GF

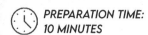 **PREPARATION TIME:**
10 MINUTES

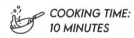 **COOKING TIME:**
10 MINUTES

 SERVING: 4
SERVING SIZE: 2 PANCAKES

Ingredients

- 1 cup almond flour
- 1/2 tsp baking powder
- 3 large eggs
- 1/4 cup unsweetened almond milk
- 1 tsp vanilla extract
- 2 tbsp sugar
- Non-stick olive oil cooking spray
- 1 cup low-sugar mixed berries

Directions

1. In a medium bowl, mix the almond flour and baking powder.
2. In another bowl, whisk together the eggs, unsweetened almond milk, vanilla extract, and sugar.
3. Combine the wet ingredients with the flour mixture until well blended. Gently fold in the mixed berries.
4. Preheat a griddle sprayed with olive oil over medium heat.
5. Pour the batter onto the skillet to form pancakes, cooking for about 2 minutes until slightly set. Flip and cook for another 2 minutes until golden brown.
6. Repeat with the remaining batter to make more pancakes. Serve warm.

Nutrition information per serving

Calories: 215; Carbs: 9g; Fat: 16g; Protein: 10g; Fiber: 4g

Slow Cooker Pear and Walnut Oatmeal | VG, EF, DF, GF

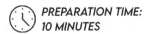 **PREPARATION TIME:**
10 MINUTES

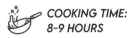 **COOKING TIME:**
8-9 HOURS

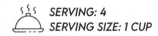 **SERVING: 4**
SERVING SIZE: 1 CUP

Ingredients

- 1 cup steel-cut oats
- 2 pears, cut into small cubes
- 1/2 cup chopped walnuts
- 4 cups water
- 2 tsp ground cinnamon
- 1/2 tsp pure vanilla extract
- 1/3 tsp ground cloves (optional)

Directions

1. Combine all ingredients in a slow cooker. Mix so ingredients are evenly distributed.
2. Set the slow cooker on a low setting, cover, and cook for 8 to 9 hours.
3. Spoon into 4 serving bowls.
4. (Optional) Serve with a splash of milk (or milk alternative), if desired.

Nutrition information per serving
Calories: 280; Fat: 12g; Carbs: 42g; Fiber: 7g; Protein: 8g

Broccoli & Swiss Cheese Egg Cups | V, GF

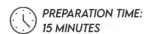 **PREPARATION TIME:**
15 MINUTES

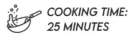 **COOKING TIME:**
25 MINUTES

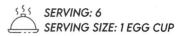 **SERVING: 6**
SERVING SIZE: 1 EGG CUP

Ingredients

- 6 large eggs
- 1 cup broccoli florets, steamed and chopped
- 1/2 cup low-sodium Swiss cheese, shredded
- 1/4 cup unsweetened almond milk
- 1/4 tsp garlic powder
- 1/4 tsp onion powder
- Pinch of black pepper

Directions

1. Preheat your oven to 375°F (190°C).
2. Grease a 6-cup muffin tin with non-stick cooking spray.
3. In a medium bowl, whisk together the eggs, unsweetened almond milk, garlic powder, onion powder, and black pepper until well combined.
4. Evenly distribute the steamed and chopped broccoli among the muffin cups.
5. Pour the egg mixture over the broccoli in each muffin cup.
6. Sprinkle the shredded low-sodium Swiss cheese on top of each egg cup.
7. Bake for 25 minutes, or until the tops are slightly golden.
8. Remove from the oven and allow to cool before removing from the muffin tin. Serve and enjoy.

Nutrition information per serving
Calories: 125; Carbs: 3g; Fat: 8g; Protein: 10g; Fiber: 1g

Shakshuka: Spicy Tomatoes and Eggs | V, DF, NF

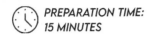 **PREPARATION TIME:** 15 MINUTES

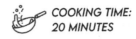 **COOKING TIME:** 20 MINUTES

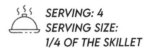 **SERVING: 4** SERVING SIZE: 1/4 OF THE SKILLET

Ingredients

- 2 tbsp olive oil
- 1 yellow onion, finely chopped
- 1 clove garlic, finely chopped
- 1 tsp ground cumin
- Kosher salt and pepper to taste
- 1 lb tomatoes, halved if large
- 8 large eggs
- 1/4 cup baby spinach, finely chopped
- Whole grain bread slices, for serving

Directions

1. Preheat your oven to 400°F. Heat olive oil in a large oven-safe skillet over medium heat. Add onion and sauté until golden brown and tender, about 8 minutes.
2. Stir in garlic, cumin, and ½ tsp each of salt and pepper, and cook for 1 minute. Add tomatoes and transfer to the oven. Roast for 10 minutes.
3. Remove the skillet from the oven, stir the tomato mixture, then make 8 small wells in the vegetables. Carefully crack an egg into each well. Return to the oven and bake until the eggs are cooked to your liking, about 7 to 8 minutes for slightly runny yolks.
4. Sprinkle with chopped spinach and, if desired, serve with slices of whole grain bread on the side.

Nutrition information per serving

Calories: 235; Carbs: 8g; Fat: 16.5g; Protein: 14g; Fiber: 2g

Cottage Cheese and Tomato Toast | V, EF, NF

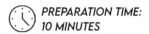 **PREPARATION TIME:**
10 MINUTES

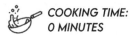 **COOKING TIME:**
0 MINUTES

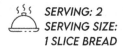 **SERVING: 2**
SERVING SIZE:
1 SLICE BREAD

Ingredients

- 2 slices of whole wheat or grain bread (low-sodium), toasted
- 1/2 cup low-fat, low-sodium cottage cheese
- 1 medium-sized tomato, sliced
- 5 leaves of fresh basil
- A pinch of black pepper

Directions

1. Spread the cottage cheese evenly on each slice of toasted bread.
2. Arrange the tomato slices over the cottage cheese on each slice.
3. Garnish with fresh basil leaves and sprinkle a pinch of black pepper over the top. Serve immediately.

Nutrition information per serving
Calories: 120; Carbs: 18g; Fat: 2g; Protein: 7g; Fiber: 3g

Green Smoothie Bowl with Berries | VG, EF, DF, GF, NF

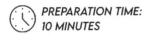 **PREPARATION TIME:**
10 MINUTES

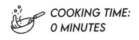 **COOKING TIME:**
0 MINUTES

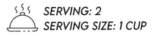 **SERVING: 2**
SERVING SIZE: 1 CUP

Ingredients

- 1 cup baby spinach
- 1/2 ripe avocado
- 1/2 cup frozen cauliflower
- 1/2 cup unsweetened coconut milk
- 1/4 cup water
- 2 tbsp chia seeds
- 1/4 tsp cinnamon
- 1/2 cup mixed berries (strawberries, raspberries, blueberries)

Directions

1. Combine baby spinach, ripe avocado, frozen cauliflower, coconut milk, water, and cinnamon in your blender. Blend until the mixture reaches a smooth consistency.
2. Add chia seeds to the blended mixture and stir well to incorporate.
3. Evenly divide the smoothie mixture into two bowls.
4. Garnish each bowl with the mixed berries before serving.

Nutrition information per serving
Calories: 215; Carbs: 17g; Fat: 14g; Protein: 6g; Fiber: 9g

LUNCH & DINNER RECIPES

Fish Mains

Citrus-Poached Sole filet | EF, DF, GF, NF

 PREPARATION TIME:
15 MINUTES

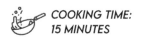 **COOKING TIME:**
15 MINUTES

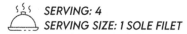 **SERVING: 4**
SERVING SIZE: 1 SOLE FILET

Ingredients

- 4 sole filets (about 6 oz each), pat dried
- 1 lemon, zested & juiced
- 1 orange, zested & juiced
- 1 lime, zested & juiced
- 1 cup low-sodium vegetable broth
- 1 tbsp olive oil
- Salt & pepper, to taste

Directions

1. Season the sole filets with salt and pepper to taste.
2. In a medium saucepan, combine the lemon, orange, and lime zests and juices with the vegetable broth. Bring to a simmer over medium heat.
3. Stir the olive oil into the citrus broth mixture until well combined.
4. Gently place the sole filets into the simmering broth. Allow them to simmer for about 7 minutes, carefully turning the filets once, until the fish is opaque and cooked through.
5. Using a spatula, carefully remove the cooked sole filets from the saucepan and transfer them to serving plates.
6. Spoon a portion of the poaching liquid over each filet before serving.

Nutrition information per serving
Calories: 228; Carbs: 9g; Fat: 6g; Protein: 33g; Fiber: 2g

Tuna Croquettes with Dill and Lemon | DF, NF

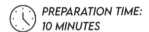 **PREPARATION TIME:** 10 MINUTES

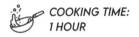 **COOKING TIME:** 1 HOUR

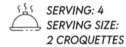 **SERVING:** 4
SERVING SIZE: 2 CROQUETTES

Ingredients

- 2 cans (5 oz each) chunk light tuna in water, drained and flaked
- 1 large russet potato (10 oz), peeled, cubed (9 oz after peeling)
- 1/4 cup chopped dill
- 2 tbsp light mayonnaise
- 2 tbsp minced red onion
- 1 tbsp mustard
- 1 tsp fresh lemon juice
- 3/4 tsp kosher salt
- Black pepper, to taste
- Olive oil spray
- 1 large egg, beaten
- 3/4 cup plain or gluten-free panko breadcrumbs
- Lemon wedges, for serving
- Tartar sauce, optional for serving

Directions

1. Place the potato cubes in a small saucepan and cover with water. Cook over medium-high heat until the potatoes are tender, about 15 minutes, then drain.
2. In a large basin, mash the boiled potatoes. Mix in tuna, dill, mayonnaise, red onion, mustard, lemon juice, salt, and black pepper. Place the mixture in the freezer for 10 minutes to harden up.
3. Form the mixture into eight logs, each with a full 1/4 cup of the mixture.
4. Dip the croquettes in the beaten egg, then coat evenly with the panko breadcrumbs. Set aside on a board. Spray olive oil on both sides of each croquette.
5. Air fried for 10 minutes at 350°F, flipping halfway through, or until golden and crispy.
6. Bake at 375°F for 20 to 25 minutes, flipping halfway through, until golden and crispy.
7. Serve the croquettes with lemon wedges and tartar sauce, if desired.

Nutrition information per serving
Calories: 215; Carbs: 21g; Fat: 4g; Protein: 23g; Fiber: 2g

Creamy Spinach-Artichoke Salmon | EF, HF, GF, NF

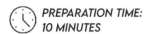 **PREPARATION TIME:**
10 MINUTES

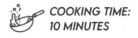 **COOKING TIME:**
10 MINUTES

SERVING: 4
SERVING SIZE: 1 SALMON
PORTION WITH SAUCE

Ingredients

- 1 1/4 pounds salmon filet, cut into 4 equal portions
- 1/2 tsp salt, divided
- 1/2 tsp ground pepper, divided
- 1 tbsp extra-virgin olive oil
- 1/4 cup shallot, halved and thinly sliced
- 1/2 cup heavy cream
- 1/4 cup low-sodium chicken broth
- 1 tsp cornstarch
- 1/4 tsp garlic powder
- 3 cups baby spinach, coarsely chopped
- 1/2 cup marinated artichoke hearts, sliced

Directions

1. Arrange a rack in the upper third of the oven. Preheat the broiler to high. Line a rimmed baking sheet with foil.
2. Place the salmon skin-side down on the prepared baking sheet. Sprinkle with 1/4 tsp each of salt and pepper. Broil for 8 to 10 minutes, rotating once from front to back, until the centre is opaque.
3. Meanwhile, heat the olive oil in a large skillet over medium-high heat. Add the shallot and cook, stirring, for 1 minute.
4. Whisk together the cream, broth, cornstarch, garlic powder, and the remaining 1/4 tsp each of salt and pepper in a measuring cup. Add to the skillet and cook, stirring, until starting to thicken, about 2 minutes.
5. Add the spinach and artichoke hearts to the skillet; cook, stirring, until the spinach has wilted, 1 to 2 minutes more.
6. Remove the skin from the salmon, if desired, and serve topped with the sauce.

Nutrition information per serving
Calories: 373; Carbs: 7g; Fat: 24g; Protein: 31g; Fiber: 2g

Honey-Ginger Grilled Sardines | EF, DF, GF, NF

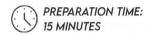 **PREPARATION TIME:** 15 MINUTES

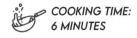 **COOKING TIME:** 6 MINUTES

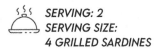 **SERVING: 2**
SERVING SIZE: 4 GRILLED SARDINES

Ingredients

- 8 fresh sardines, cleaned and gutted
- 2 tbsp low-sodium soy sauce
- 2 tbsp honey
- 1 tbsp grated ginger
- Juice of 1 lemon
- 2 cloves garlic, minced
- Ground black pepper, to taste
- Non-stick cooking olive oil spray

Directions

1. Preheat your grill to medium-high heat.
2. In a small bowl, whisk together soy sauce, honey, grated ginger, lemon juice, minced garlic, and black pepper.
3. Place the sardines in a shallow container, then pour the honey-ginger marinade over them. Allow marinating for 10 minutes.
4. Spray the grill grates with olive oil spray. Grill the marinated sardines for 3 minutes on each side, until cooked through. Serve.

Nutrition information per serving

Calories: 190; Carbs: 8g; Fat: 9g; Protein: 21g; Fiber: 0g

Italian Baked Shrimp with Zucchini Spaghetti

EF, DF, GF, NF

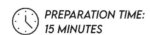 **PREPARATION TIME:** 15 MINUTES

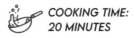 **COOKING TIME:** 20 MINUTES

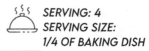 **SERVING:** 4 SERVING SIZE: 1/4 OF BAKING DISH

Ingredients

- 1-pound medium shrimp, peeled & deveined
- 4 medium zucchinis, spiralized into noodles
- 2 cups cherry tomatoes, halved
- 1/4 cup fresh basil leaves, chopped
- 1/4 cup fresh parsley leaves, chopped
- 2 cloves garlic, minced
- Juice of 1 lemon
- 1 tbsp olive oil
- Salt & ground black pepper, to taste

Directions

1. Preheat your oven to 400°F.
2. In a large bowl, mix together shrimp, cherry tomatoes, basil, parsley, garlic, lemon juice, olive oil, salt, and pepper.
3. Place the spiralized zucchini spaghetti in an oven-safe baking dish. Top with the shrimp and tomato mixture.
4. Cover the baking dish with aluminum foil and bake for 15 to 20 minutes until the shrimp are pink and fully cooked. Serve.

Nutrition information per serving

Calories: 261; Carbs: 13g; Fat: 8g; Protein: 34g; Fiber: 4g

Garlic and Lime Baked Grouper | EF, DF, GF, NF

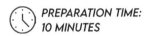 **PREPARATION TIME:** 10 MINUTES

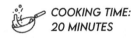 **COOKING TIME:** 20 MINUTES

 SERVING: 4
SERVING SIZE:
1 GROUPER FILET

Ingredients

- 4 grouper filets (about 6 oz each), patted dry
- 4 cloves garlic, minced
- Zest and juice of 2 limes
- 1 tbsp olive oil
- Salt and pepper, to taste
- Lime wedges, for garnish

Directions

1. Preheat Oven: Set your oven to 375°F. Prepare a baking sheet by lining it with parchment paper.
2. Lightly season the grouper filets with salt and pepper, and arrange them on the prepared baking sheet.
3. In a small bowl, combine the minced garlic, lime zest, lime juice, and olive oil. Mix well until all the ingredients are thoroughly combined.
4. Spoon the garlic and lime mixture over each grouper filet, spreading it evenly to cover the tops.
5. Place the baking sheet in the oven and bake for 15 to 20 minutes, or until the grouper flakes easily when tested with a fork.
6. Once done, remove the grouper from the oven and garnish each filet with a lime wedge. Serve hot with a side of your favorite vegetables or a fresh salad for a complete meal.

Nutrition information per serving

Calories: 240; Carbs: 4g; Fat: 7g; Protein: 40g; Fiber: <1g

Marinated Broiled Tuna Steaks | EF, DF, GF, NF

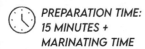 **PREPARATION TIME:**
15 MINUTES +
MARINATING TIME

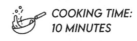 **COOKING TIME:**
10 MINUTES

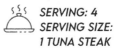 **SERVING: 4**
SERVING SIZE:
1 TUNA STEAK

Ingredients

- 4 tuna steaks (6 oz each)
- 2 tbsp lemon juice
- 2 tbsp low-sodium soy sauce
- 2 tbsp olive oil
- 1 tsp fresh ginger, grated
- 2 garlic cloves, minced
- Fresh cracked black pepper, to taste

Directions

1. In a shallow container, whisk together lemon juice, soy sauce, olive oil, grated ginger, and minced garlic. Add the tuna steaks, ensuring both sides are well coated with the marinade. Cover and refrigerate for at least 1 hour to allow the flavors to meld.
2. Turn your broiler on high heat. Line a baking sheet with aluminum foil for easy cleanup.
3. Place the marinated tuna steaks on the prepared baking sheet. Season each steak generously with fresh cracked black pepper.
4. Broil the tuna steaks 4-5 minutes per side, or until they are cooked to your desired level of doneness. Keep an eye on them to prevent overcooking.
5. Once broiled to perfection, remove the tuna steaks from the oven and serve immediately. Enjoy the rich flavors and tender texture of this exquisite seafood dish.

Nutrition information per serving

Calories: 320; Carbs: 2g; Fat: 14g; Protein: 46g; Fiber: 1g

Stuffed Eggplants with Rice | VG, EF, DF, GF, NF

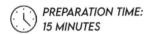 **PREPARATION TIME:**
15 MINUTES

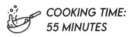 **COOKING TIME:**
55 MINUTES

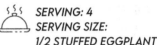 **SERVING: 4**
SERVING SIZE:
1/2 STUFFED EGGPLANT

Ingredients

- 6.3 oz basmati rice
- 2 eggplants (26.5 oz total)
- 2.8 oz cooked chickpeas
- 1/2 red onion
- 1 oz olives
- 6 sun-dried tomatoes
- 1 tbsp capers
- 1/2 tsp oregano
- 1 tsp marjoram
- 1 tsp chopped dill
- Olive oil for drizzling
- Salt to taste

Directions

1. Preheat your oven to 392°F (200°C). Cut the eggplants in half lengthwise and make shallow cuts in the flesh. Season with salt and olive oil. Bake for 25 minutes until softened. Scoop out some of the flesh to create a hollow.
2. Cook the basmati rice in boiling salted water until al dente, then drain.
3. In a skillet, sauté the chopped onion with a splash of olive oil, a pinch of salt, oregano, and marjoram for 10 minutes until softened. After 5 minutes, add the chickpeas, capers, olives, and chopped sun-dried tomatoes. Finally, add the rice and dill and cook for another couple of minutes to blend the flavors.
4. Fill each eggplant half with the rice mixture, drizzle with a bit more olive oil, and bake at 356°F (180°C) for 10-15 minutes. Serve warm or at room temperature.

Nutrition information per serving

Calories: 280; Carbs: 45g; Fat: 5g; Protein: 8g; Fiber: 7g

Grilled Veggie & White Bean Whole Wheat Wrap

VG, EF, DF, HF, NF

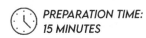 **PREPARATION TIME:** 15 MINUTES

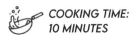 **COOKING TIME:** 10 MINUTES

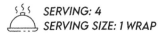 **SERVING: 4** SERVING SIZE: 1 WRAP

Ingredients

- 4 large whole wheat tortillas, warmed
- 1 cup cooked white bean, rinsed and drained
- 1 small zucchini, thinly sliced lengthwise
- 1 small yellow squash, thinly sliced lengthwise
- 1 small red bell pepper, thinly sliced
- 1 small red onion, thinly sliced
- 2 cups baby spinach leaves
- 4 tbsp lemon-tahini dressing (see recipe below)
- Olive oil spray

For the Lemon-Tahini Dressing:

- 1/4 cup tahini
- 2 tbsp fresh lemon juice
- 1 tbsp apple cider vinegar
- 1 tbsp water
- Salt & pepper, as required

Directions

1. Preheat your grill over medium-high heat.
2. Whisk all lemon-tahini dressing ingredients in a bowl, then season with salt and pepper. Set aside.
3. Lightly spray zucchini, squash, bell pepper, and onion slices with olive oil spray, then place them on the grill.
4. Cook for about 5 minutes on each side until slightly charred. Remove.
5. Assemble wraps by evelyn placing baby spinach leaves in each tortilla, followed by grilled vegetables and chickpeas. Drizzle with lemon-tahini dressing.
6. Roll up the tortillas tightly to secure the filling inside.

Nutrition information per serving

Calories: 350; Carbs: 52g; Fat: 12g; Protein: 14g; Fiber: 9g

Bean and Spinach Rice Casserole
VG, EF, DF, HF, GF, NF

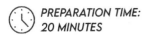 **PREPARATION TIME:**
20 MINUTES

 **COOKING TIME:**
45 MINUTES

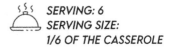 **SERVING: 6**
SERVING SIZE:
1/6 OF THE CASSEROLE

Ingredients

- 2 cups cooked brown rice
- 1 cup canned black beans, rinsed & drained
- 1 cup chopped fresh spinach
- 1 medium onion, finely chopped
- 1/2 cup low-sodium vegetable broth
- 3 cloves garlic, minced
- 2 tsp chili powder
- 1 tsp ground cumin
- Salt & pepper to taste
- Non-stick cooking olive oil spray

Directions

1. Preheat your oven to 375°F. Lightly coat a small baking dish with non-stick cooking spray.
2. In a microwave-safe bowl, mix onion, garlic, and broth. Microwave on high for about 3 minutes until onions are softened.
3. Mix cooked brown rice, black beans, chopped spinach, cooked onion and garlic mixture, chili powder, cumin, salt, and pepper in a large bowl.
4. Transfer the mixture to the prepared baking dish, pressing it down.
5. Bake the casserole for about 45 minutes until it is heated through.
6. Cool it down, slice, then serve.

Nutrition information per serving
Calories: 195; Carbs: 38g; Fat: 2g; Protein: 7g; Fiber: 8g

Baked Tofu in Parchment | VG, EF, DF, GF, NF

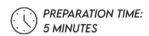 **PREPARATION TIME:**
5 MINUTES

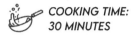 **COOKING TIME:**
30 MINUTES

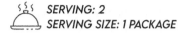 **SERVING: 2**
SERVING SIZE: 1 PACKAGE

Ingredients

- 7 oz tofu
- 12 black olives
- 2 tbsp capers
- 8 cherry tomatoes
- 1 shallot, thinly sliced
- 2 tbsp extra-virgin olive oil
- 2 pinches sea salt
- 2 pinches black pepper
- 1 tsp dried oregano
- 1 tsp lemon thyme
- 1 tbsp sunflower seeds

Directions

1. Blanch the tofu blocks in boiling salted water for 2 minutes to remove bitterness. Drain and cut into 0.8-inch cubes.
2. In a bowl, mix the tofu cubes with olives, capers, oregano, lemon thyme, cherry tomatoes, sunflower seeds, and sliced shallot. Season with salt, pepper, and drizzle with olive oil.
3. Lay out two rectangles of parchment paper. Divide the mixture between the two sheets, placing it in the center. Fold the parchment paper over the mixture, sealing the edges to form a parcel.
4. Bake in a preheated oven at 356°F with fan mode for about 30 minutes.
5. Serve the parcels hot, allowing guests to open them and enjoy the steamy, aromatic contents.
6. The tofu can be marinated beforehand to enhance its flavor. Vary the vegetables according to the season for different flavors.

Nutrition information per serving

Calories: 210; Carbs: 8g; Fat: 16g; Protein: 12g; Fiber: 3g

Tempeh Ratatouille on Whole Grain Rice

VG, EF, DF, GF, NF

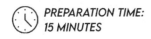 **PREPARATION TIME:** 15 MINUTES

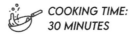 **COOKING TIME:** 30 MINUTES

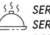 **SERVING: 4** SERVING SIZE: 1/4 OF THE POT + 1/2 CUP RICE

Ingredients

- 1 medium zucchini, thinly sliced
- 1 medium yellow squash, thinly sliced
- 1 small eggplant, thinly sliced
- 1 medium red bell pepper, chopped
- 1 medium onion, chopped
- 2 garlic cloves, minced
- 1 (14.5 oz) can no-salt-added diced tomatoes, drained
- 8 oz tempeh, cubed
- 2 cups cooked brown rice
- 2 tbsp fresh basil, chopped
- 1 tbsp fresh oregano, chopped
- 3 tbsp balsamic vinegar
- Salt & pepper, to taste

Directions

1. Over medium heat, cook onions in a large non-stick pot until translucent, about 5 minutes. Add garlic; cook for 1 minute, stirring frequently.
2. Incorporate zucchini, yellow squash, and balsamic vinegar; cook covered on low heat for 5 minutes.
3. Add tempeh and eggplant; cover and cook for 10 minutes until vegetables are soft.
4. Stir in tomatoes, red bell pepper, basil, and oregano. Cook covered on low-medium heat for another 10 minutes or until all vegetables are tender. Season with salt and pepper.
5. Serve the ratatouille over brown rice, garnishing with additional fresh herbs if desired.

Nutrition information per serving

Calories: 390; Carbs: 58g; Fat: 11g; Protein: 20g; Fiber: 9g

Baked Zucchini Parmesan Casserole | V, EF, GF

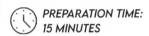 **PREPARATION TIME:**
15 MINUTES

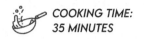 **COOKING TIME:**
35 MINUTES

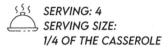 **SERVING: 4**
SERVING SIZE:
1/4 OF THE CASSEROLE

Ingredients

- 4 medium zucchinis, thinly sliced
- 1/2 cup grated Parmesan cheese
- 1 cup low-fat mozzarella cheese, shredded
- 1/4 cup almond flour
- 1/2 tsp garlic powder
- 1/2 tsp dried basil
- 1/2 tsp dried oregano
- Salt & pepper, to taste
- Non-stick cooking olive oil spray

Directions

1. Preheat your oven to 350°F. Spray a medium-sized baking dish with non-stick cooking spray.
2. In a small bowl, mix almond flour, garlic powder, basil, oregano, salt, and pepper.
3. Begin with a layer of sliced zucchini in the prepared baking dish. Sprinkle a third of the Parmesan cheese and a third of the almond flour mixture on top.
4. Add another layer of zucchini, followed by another third of the Parmesan cheese and almond flour mixture. Repeat for another layer.
5. Top with shredded mozzarella cheese as the final layer.
6. Bake for 35 minutes or until the cheese is bubbly and golden. Allow to cool slightly before serving.

Nutrition information per serving

Calories: 150; Carbs: 10g; Fat: 8g; Protein: 11g; Fiber: 3g

Eggplant Rollatini with Ricotta | V, EF, HF, GF

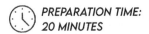 **PREPARATION TIME:**
20 MINUTES

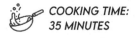 **COOKING TIME:**
35 MINUTES

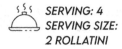 **SERVING: 4**
SERVING SIZE:
2 ROLLATINI

Ingredients

- 2 large eggplants, sliced lengthwise into 1/4-inch-thick slices (about 16 slices total)
- Olive oil cooking spray
- 1 cup homemade marinara sauce (low-sodium & low-sugar), divided
- 2 cups traditional ricotta cheese
- 1/4 cup nutritional yeast
- 2 cups fresh spinach leaves, chopped
- 1/4 tsp black pepper

Directions

1. Preheat the oven to 375°F. Line a baking sheet with parchment paper and spray with olive oil cooking spray.
2. Arrange eggplant slices on the prepared baking sheet. Lightly spray the eggplant slices with olive oil.
3. Bake the eggplant slices for 15 minutes, or until they are tender. Remove from the oven and allow to cool slightly.
4. In a bowl, mix traditional ricotta cheese, nutritional yeast, spinach, and black pepper.
5. Spread half of the marinara sauce on the bottom of a baking dish.
6. Place a heaping spoonful of the ricotta-spinach mixture on one end of each eggplant slice, then roll it up tightly.
7. Arrange the rolls seam side down in the baking dish. Repeat with the remaining eggplant slices and filling.
8. Pour the remaining marinara sauce over the top of the eggplant rolls.
9. Bake for 20 minutes, or until heated through. Remove from the oven and let cool slightly before serving.

Nutrition information per serving
Calories: 275; Carbs: 25g; Fat: 11g; Protein: 17g; Fiber: 8g

Baked Turkey & Spinach Meatballs | GF

PREPARATION TIME:
15 MINUTES

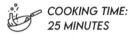

COOKING TIME:
25 MINUTES

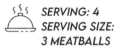

SERVING: 4
SERVING SIZE:
3 MEATBALLS

Ingredients

- 1 pound lean ground turkey
- 2 cups fresh spinach, finely chopped
- 1/4 cup low-fat feta cheese, crumbled
- 1/4 cup almond flour
- 1 large egg, beaten
- 1/2 onion, diced
- 2 cloves garlic, minced
- 1 tbsp low-sodium Italian seasoning
- Cooking spray

Directions

1. Preheat your oven to 400°F. In a large bowl, combine the ground turkey, spinach, feta cheese, almond flour, beaten egg, onion, garlic, and Italian seasoning.
2. Line a baking sheet with parchment paper and lightly spray with cooking spray.
3. Form the mixture into meatballs and place them on the prepared baking sheet.
4. Bake for 20 to 25 minutes, until the meatballs are cooked through. Remove from the oven and allow to cool slightly before serving.

Nutrition information per serving

Calories: 250; Carbs: 6g; Fat: 12g; Protein: 30g; Fiber: 2g

Broccoli & Chicken Rice Skillet | EF, GF NF

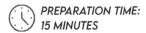 **PREPARATION TIME:**
15 MINUTES

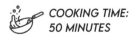 **COOKING TIME:**
50 MINUTES

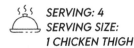 **SERVING: 4**
SERVING SIZE:
1 CHICKEN THIGH

Ingredients

- 2 1/4 cups reduced-sodium chicken broth
- 2 tbsp lemon juice
- 1 tbsp Dijon mustard
- 1 tsp chopped fresh oregano, plus more for garnish
- 2 tbsp extra-virgin olive oil, divided
- 3/4 tsp salt, divided
- 1/2 tsp ground pepper, divided
- 4 bone-in, skin-on chicken thighs
- 1 small head broccoli (about 16 oz), cut into 6 (1 1/2- to 2-inch-thick) wedges
- 1 cup brown basmati rice
- 1/4 cup crumbled feta cheese
- Lemon wedges for serving (optional)

Directions

1. Preheat the oven to 350° F. In a medium bowl, whisk together the broth, lemon juice, mustard, oregano, 1 tbsp oil, 1/2 tsp salt, and 1/4 tsp pepper.
2. Sprinkle the chicken with the remaining 1/4 tsp of salt and pepper. Heat the remaining 1 tbsp oil in a large oven-safe skillet over medium-high heat. Cook the chicken, skin side down, until golden brown and crispy, about 6 minutes. Transfer to a plate.
3. Cook the broccoli wedges in the pan over medium-high heat, flipping once, until slightly browned and tender, about 2 to 3 minutes per side. Transfer to a different plate.
4. Reduce the heat to medium and cook the rice, stirring constantly, until toasted and aromatic, about 1 minute. Stir in the broth mixture until well mixed.
5. Place the broccoli wedges and chicken, skin side up, in the rice mixture. Bring to a boil over medium high heat. Cover with a tightly fitted lid.
6. Bake for 45 minutes, or until the liquid has been absorbed, the rice is soft, and a thermometer inserted into the chicken reads at least 165°F. Remove the lid and bake for 5 minutes, or until the chicken skins are somewhat crispy.
7. Remove from the oven and evenly sprinkle with feta. Garnish with oregano and serve with lemon wedges as preferred.

Nutrition information per serving

Calories: 418; Carbs: 40g; Fat: 17g; Protein: 28g; Fiber: 5g

Creamy Sun-Dried Tomato and Shallot Chicken
EF, GF, NF

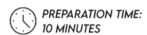 **PREPARATION TIME:**
10 MINUTES

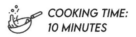 **COOKING TIME:**
10 MINUTES

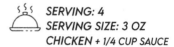 **SERVING: 4**
SERVING SIZE: 3 OZ
CHICKEN + 1/4 CUP SAUCE

Ingredients

- 1 pound chicken cutlets
- 1/4 tsp salt, divided
- 1/4 tsp ground pepper, divided
- 1/2 cup slivered oil-packed sun-dried tomatoes, plus 1 tbsp oil from the jar
- 1/2 cup finely chopped shallots
- 1/2 cup dry white wine
- 1/2 cup heavy cream
- 2 tbsp chopped fresh parsley

Directions

1. Sprinkle the chicken with 1/8 tsp salt and pepper. Heat the sun-dried tomato oil in a large skillet over medium heat. Cook the chicken, rotating once, until browned and an instant-read thermometer put into the thickest section reads 165°F, about 6 minutes total. Transfer to a plate.
2. Add the sun-dried tomatoes and shallots to the pan. Cook, stirring, for one minute. Increase the heat to high and add the wine. Cook, scraping up any browned parts, until most of the liquid has evaporated, about 2 minutes.
3. Reduce the heat to medium, then pour in the cream, any collected chicken juices, and the remaining 1/8 tsp salt and pepper; simmer for 2 minutes. Return the chicken to the pan and turn to coat in the sauce. Serve the chicken topped with the sauce and parsley.

Nutrition information per serving
Calories: 324; Carbs: 8g; Fat: 19g; Protein: 25g; Fiber: 1g

Italian Chicken & Veggie Casserole | EF, DF, GF, NF

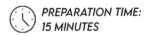 **PREPARATION TIME:**
15 MINUTES

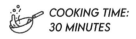 **COOKING TIME:**
30 MINUTES

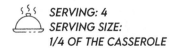 **SERVING: 4**
SERVING SIZE:
1/4 OF THE CASSEROLE

Ingredients

- 16 oz boneless, skinless chicken breast, cubed
- 2 medium zucchini, thinly sliced
- 1 red bell pepper, chopped
- 1 yellow bell pepper, chopped
- 1 cup cherry tomatoes, halved
- 1/2 onion, chopped
- 3 cloves garlic, minced
- 2 tbsp olive oil
- 1 tsp dried basil
- 1 tsp dried oregano
- 1/4 tsp black pepper

Directions

1. Preheat your oven to 375°F.
2. In a large bowl, combine chicken, zucchini, bell peppers, cherry tomatoes, onion, and garlic.
3. In a small bowl, mix olive oil, basil, oregano, and black pepper. Pour over the chicken and vegetables; toss until well coated.
4. Spread the chicken and vegetable mixture in a large 9x13-inch casserole dish.
5. Bake for 30 minutes, until the chicken is cooked through. Remove from the oven and let it rest for a few minutes before serving.

Nutrition information per serving
Calories: 295; Carbs: 12g; Fat: 11g; Protein: 37g; Fiber: 3g

Prosciutto, Mozzarella, and Melon Salad | EF, GF, NF

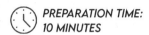 **PREPARATION TIME:** 10 MINUTES

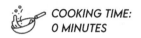 **COOKING TIME:** 0 MINUTES

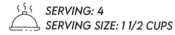 **SERVING: 4** SERVING SIZE: 1 1/2 CUPS

Ingredients

For the dressing:

- 1 tbsp extra virgin olive oil
- 1 tbsp balsamic vinegar
- 1/2 tbsp fresh squeezed lemon juice
- 1/8 tsp kosher salt
- Fresh black pepper, to taste

For the Salad:

- 5 cups baby arugula
- 4 ripe melon slices, cut into bite-sized pieces
- 4 oz fresh mozzarella, sliced and torn into pieces
- 2 oz thin sliced prosciutto, torn into pieces

Directions

1. In a small bowl, whisk together the olive oil, balsamic vinegar, lemon juice, salt, and black pepper to create the dressing.
2. On a large serving platter, arrange the baby arugula as the base layer.
3. Distribute the torn pieces of prosciutto evenly over the arugula.
4. Scatter the melon pieces and torn fresh mozzarella across the salad.
5. Add fresh basil or mint leaves for garnish (optional)
6. Right before serving, drizzle the prepared dressing over the salad, ensuring all ingredients are lightly coated.

Nutrition information per serving

Calories: 196; Carbs: 12g; Fat: 12.5g; Protein: 10g; Fiber: 2g

Rosemary Garlic Lamb Loin Chops | EF, DF, GF, NF

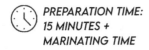 **PREPARATION TIME:**
15 MINUTES +
MARINATING TIME

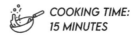 **COOKING TIME:**
15 MINUTES

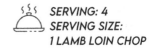 **SERVING: 4**
SERVING SIZE:
1 LAMB LOIN CHOP

Ingredients

- 4 lamb loin chops (approximately 6 oz each)
- 2 tbsp fresh rosemary, finely chopped
- 4 garlic cloves, minced
- 2 tbsp olive oil
- 1/2 tsp black pepper
- 1 lemon, zested and juiced
- Salt-free seasoning blend (optional)

Directions

1. In a small bowl, combine the rosemary, garlic, olive oil, black pepper, lemon zest, and lemon juice to create the marinade.
2. Place the lamb loin chops in a shallow dish. Pour the marinade over the chops, ensuring they are well coated. Cover the dish and let the chops marinate in the refrigerator for at least 1 hour.
3. Preheat your oven to 400°F (200°C). Line a baking sheet with aluminum foil and place a wire rack on top.
4. Arrange the marinated lamb chops on the wire rack. If desired, sprinkle with a salt-free seasoning blend for additional flavor.
5. Bake in the preheated oven for approximately 15 minutes, or until the chops reach your desired level of doneness. For medium-rare, an internal temperature of 145°F (63°C) is recommended.
6. Remove the chops from the oven and let them rest for a few minutes before serving. This allows the juices to redistribute throughout the meat.

Nutrition information per serving

Calories: 364; Carbs: 3g; Fat: 23g; Protein: 33g; Fiber: 0.5g

PASTA & SOUP RECIPES

Pasta

Whole Wheat Spaghetti with Vegetable Pesto
VG, EF, DF, HF

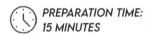 *PREPARATION TIME:*
15 MINUTES

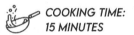 *COOKING TIME:*
15 MINUTES

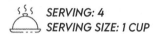 *SERVING: 4*
SERVING SIZE: 1 CUP

Ingredients

- 8 oz whole wheat spaghetti
- 2 cups fresh basil leaves, packed
- 1 cup baby spinach
- 1/2 cup cherry tomatoes, halved
- 1/4 cup pine nuts, toasted
- 2 garlic cloves, minced
- Salt & pepper, to taste

Directions

1. Boil a large pot of water. Add the whole wheat spaghetti and cook until tender. Strain and set aside.
2. In a food processor, combine basil leaves, spinach, pine nuts, garlic, salt, and pepper. Process until smooth.
3. Add the cherry tomatoes to the food processor and pulse until well combined but still chunky for texture.
4. In a large bowl, toss the cooked spaghetti with the vegetable pesto until evenly coated.
5. Divide the spaghetti evenly among four plates. Serve immediately.

Nutrition information per serving
Calories: 375; Carbs: 55g; Fat: 10g; Protein: 16g; Fiber: 8g

Light Italian Carbonara | NF

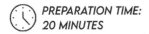 **PREPARATION TIME:**
20 MINUTES

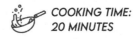 **COOKING TIME:**
20 MINUTES

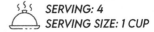 **SERVING: 4**
SERVING SIZE: 1 CUP

Ingredients

- 8 oz whole-wheat spaghetti
- 8 oz shredded cooked chicken breast
- 4 large egg yolks
- 1/2 cup grated Pecorino Romano cheese, divided
- 1/2 tsp ground pepper, plus more for garnish
- 1/4 tsp salt

Directions

1. Bring a large pot of water to a boil. Add pasta and cook according to package directions.
2. Place shredded cooked chicken in a large, warm skillet to heat through, stirring occasionally, for about 1 minute. Remove from heat.
3. Whisk egg yolks, 1/4 cup cheese, pepper, and salt together in a large heatproof metal bowl. Using tongs, transfer the cooked pasta directly from the boiling water to the bowl with the egg yolk mixture; toss gently until the cheese melts, about 30 seconds.
4. Place the bowl with the pasta over the pot with the boiling water; cook, stirring constantly, until the sauce thickens and coats the pasta, about 1 minute. Remove the bowl from the pot; stir in the warmed chicken.
5. Divide the pasta into four dishes and top with the remaining 1/4 cup cheese. If desired, garnish with more pepper.

Nutrition information per serving
Calories: 460; Carbs: 43g; Fat: 17g; Protein: 34g; Fiber: 5g

Pea Pasta, Roasted Vegetables & Arugula Pesto

V, EF, HF, GF

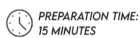 **PREPARATION TIME:** 15 MINUTES

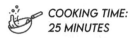 **COOKING TIME:** 25 MINUTES

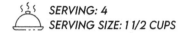 **SERVING:** 4 SERVING SIZE: 1 1/2 CUPS

Ingredients

- 8 oz pea pasta (or whole wheat pasta)
- 2 medium zucchinis, cut into thin rounds
- 1 large red bell pepper, cut into thin strips
- 1 tbsp olive oil
- Salt & pepper, as required
- 1 cup cherry tomatoes, halved

For Arugula Pesto:
- 2 cups fresh arugula, packed
- 1/2 cup fresh basil leaves, packed
- 1/3 cup pine nuts (or walnuts)
- 1/2 cup extra-virgin olive oil
- 2 cloves garlic, minced
- 1/2 cup grated Parmesan cheese (or nutritional yeast for VG version)
- Juice of 1 lemon
- Salt and pepper, to taste

Directions

1. Preheat your oven to 400°F. Toss the zucchini slices and red bell pepper strips with olive oil, salt, and pepper. Arrange them on a lined baking sheet.
2. Roast the vegetables for about 20 minutes until tender.
3. Boil your large pot with water. Add the pea pasta and cook according to the package instructions until tender. Strain, then rinse under cold water.
4. Make the Arugula Pesto by combining the arugula, basil leaves, pine nuts, garlic, olive oil, Parmesan cheese (or nutritional yeast), and lemon juice in a food processor. Process until smooth, then season with salt and pepper to taste.
5. Combine the cooked pea pasta, roasted vegetables, cherry tomatoes, and homemade arugula pesto in a large bowl. Toss everything together until the pasta and vegetables are evenly coated with the pesto.
6. Divide the mixture equally among four plates or bowls. Serve immediately.

Nutrition information per serving

Calories: 320; Carbs: 46g; Fat: 9g; Protein: 15g; Fiber: 8g

Whole Wheat Linguine with Mushroom Ragu

V, EF, HF

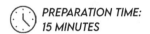 **PREPARATION TIME:** 15 MINUTES   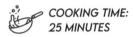 **COOKING TIME:** 25 MINUTES   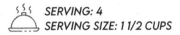 **SERVING: 4** SERVING SIZE: 1 1/2 CUPS

Ingredients

- 8 oz whole wheat linguine
- 1 tbsp olive oil
- 1 small yellow onion, chopped
- 2 cloves garlic, minced
- 16 oz assorted fresh mushrooms, sliced
- 1 (14.5 oz) can low-sodium diced tomatoes, drained
- 1/4 cup vegetable broth
- 1/2 cup homemade basil pesto sauce
- 1/4 tsp black pepper

Directions

1. Boil your large pot with water. Add the whole wheat linguine and cook until tender. Strain, then put aside.
2. Heat the olive oil in a large skillet over medium heat. Add the chopped onion and cook for about 5 minutes until softened. Add garlic and cook for about 1 minute.
3. Increase the heat to medium-high and add the sliced mushrooms. Cook for about 8 minutes until tender.
4. Add the drained diced tomatoes and vegetable broth, then bring to a simmer. Reduce the heat to low and simmer for about 10 minutes until the mixture has slightly thickened.
5. Stir in the homemade basil pesto sauce and black pepper. Toss the sauce with the cooked whole wheat linguine.
6. Serve hot and enjoy a delicious and hearty meal.

Nutrition information per serving

Calories: 389; Carbs: 63g; Fat: 10g; Protein: 19g; Fiber: 11g

Creamy Mushroom Pasta | V, EF, NF

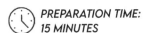 **PREPARATION TIME:**
15 MINUTES

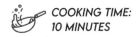 **COOKING TIME:**
10 MINUTES

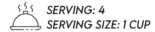 **SERVING: 4**
SERVING SIZE: 1 CUP

Ingredients

- 9 oz of whole grain pasta
- 2 tbsp olive oil
- 1 small onion, finely chopped
- 17 oz mixed mushrooms, sliced
- 2 tbsp tomato paste
- 1 cup heavy cream
- Salt and pepper, to taste
- 1/4 cup grated Parmesan cheese
- 2 tbsp chopped fresh parsley

Directions

1. Cook pasta according to package instructions until al dente. Drain and set aside.
2. In a large skillet over medium heat, heat olive oil. Add the onion and sauté until soft and translucent.
3. Add the mushrooms to the skillet and cook until they release their moisture and start to brown.
4. Stir in the tomato paste and cook for another minute.
5. Pour in the heavy cream, reduce the heat, and simmer until the sauce thickens. Season with salt and pepper.
6. Add the cooked pasta to the skillet, tossing well to coat in the creamy mushroom sauce.
7. Sprinkle with Parmesan cheese and chopped parsley. Serve immediately for the best texture and flavor.

Nutrition information per serving
Calories: 450; Carbs: 50g; Fat: 20g; Protein: 15g; Fiber: 3g

Chicken-Vegetable Quinoa Stew | EF, DF, HF, GF, NF

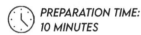 *PREPARATION TIME:*
10 MINUTES

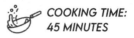 *COOKING TIME:*
45 MINUTES

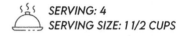 *SERVING: 4*
SERVING SIZE: 1 1/2 CUPS

Ingredients

- 1 pound boneless, skinless chicken breast, cubed
- 1 cup quinoa, rinsed and drained
- 3 cups low-sodium chicken broth
- 2 cups water
- 1 medium onion, chopped
- 2 cloves garlic, minced
- 2 carrots, peeled and sliced
- 1 zucchini, diced
- 1 red bell pepper, chopped
- 2 cups kale, stems removed and leaves chopped
- 1/4 cup fresh parsley, chopped
- Juice of one lemon
- Salt and pepper, to taste

Directions

1. In a large pot, combine onion and garlic with a bit of water over medium heat. Cook for about 5 minutes until softened.
2. Add the cubed chicken and cook for about 5 minutes until no longer pink on the outside. Add the quinoa and cook for an additional minute.
3. Pour the broth and water into the pot. Bring to a boil, then reduce to a simmer for about 15 minutes.
4. Add the carrots, zucchini, bell pepper, salt, and pepper. Continue simmering for about 10 minutes until the vegetables are tender.
5. Stir in the kale leaves and chopped parsley, then cook for another 5 minutes until the kale is wilted. Remove from heat, then stir in fresh lemon juice. Serve.

Nutrition information per serving

Calories: 375; Carbs: 47g; Fat: 6g; Protein: 36g; Fiber: 7g

Triple Mushroom Barley Soup

VG, EF, DF, HF, GF, NF

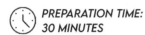 **PREPARATION TIME:**
30 MINUTES

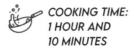 **COOKING TIME:**
1 HOUR AND
10 MINUTES

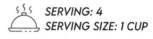 **SERVING: 4**
SERVING SIZE: 1 CUP

Ingredients

- 1/2 oz dried porcini mushrooms
- 1 large yellow onion
- 1 carrot, finely chopped
- 1 rib celery, chopped to make 1/4 cup
- 12 oz fresh mushrooms, thinly sliced
- 6 medium or large fresh shiitake mushrooms, stems removed, washed, and sliced
- 3 quarts (12 cups) vegetable stock
- 2 cups hulled barley or pearled barley
- 1 bay leaf
- 4 tbsp balsamic vinegar, or to taste
- Pepper, to taste
- Parsley or cilantro, for garnish
- 1 bag (3-4 handfuls) spinach

Directions

1. Soak the dried porcini mushrooms in warm water for about 30 minutes, or until soft. Drain and squeeze out the liquid into a bowl; reserve this liquid for later use in the soup. Roughly chop the rehydrated porcini mushrooms.
2. In a large soup pot, stir-fry the onion until it begins to soften. Add the carrots, celery, and all mushrooms. Cook for a few minutes until the fresh mushrooms begin to soften.
3. Pour in the vegetable stock, add the barley, bay leaf, and the reserved porcini soaking liquid. Bring the mixture to a boil, then reduce the heat and simmer for 1 hour, adding more liquid if necessary.
4. Season the soup with balsamic vinegar and pepper to taste. Just before serving, fold in your choice of cilantro or parsley and the spinach until the spinach wilts.

Nutrition information per serving
Calories: 180; Carbs: 36g; Fat: 1g; Protein: 6g; Fiber: 9g

Cauliflower, Fennel, and Leek Chowder

VG, EF, DF, HF, GF, NF

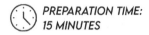 **PREPARATION TIME:** 15 MINUTES

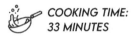 **COOKING TIME:** 33 MINUTES

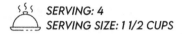 **SERVING: 4** SERVING SIZE: 1 1/2 CUPS

Ingredients

- 1 medium cauliflower head, chopped into florets
- 1 fennel bulb, thinly sliced
- 2 leeks (white & light green parts only), thinly sliced
- 1 tbsp olive oil
- 4 cups low-sodium vegetable broth
- 2 cloves garlic, minced
- 1 tsp dried thyme
- Salt & pepper, to taste

Directions

1. In a large pot, heat the olive oil over medium heat. Add the sliced leeks and cook for about 5 minutes until they become soft.
2. Add the garlic and fennel, then cook for another 3 minutes. Stir in the cauliflower florets, broth, and dried thyme. Bring to a boil.
3. Reduce to a simmer and cook for about 25 minutes until the cauliflower is tender.
4. Puree the soup using an immersion blender until your desired consistency is reached. Season with salt and pepper to taste. Serve warm.

Nutrition information per serving

Calories: 152; Carbs: 24g; Fat: 5g; Protein: 6g; Fiber: 7g

Hearty Lentil and Vegetable Soup

VG, EF, DF, HF, GF, NF

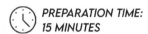 **PREPARATION TIME:**
15 MINUTES

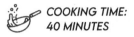 **COOKING TIME:**
40 MINUTES

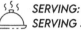 **SERVING: 4**
SERVING SIZE: 1 1/2 CUPS

Ingredients

- 1 cup green or brown lentils, washed and strained
- 4 cups low-sodium vegetable broth
- 2 cups water
- 1 medium onion, chopped
- 2 large carrots, peeled and diced
- 2 celery stalks, chopped
- 2 garlic cloves, minced
- 1 medium zucchini, diced
- 1 red bell pepper, diced
- 1 (14.5 oz) can no-salt-added diced tomatoes, drained
- 1 bay leaf
- 1/2 tsp dried thyme
- Ground black pepper, to taste

Directions

1. In a large pot, bring the lentils, broth, and water to a boil over medium-high heat. Reduce to low heat and simmer for 15 minutes.
2. Stir in the onion, carrots, celery, garlic, zucchini, red bell pepper, diced tomatoes, bay leaf, dried thyme, and black pepper.
3. Continue to simmer the soup for an additional 25 minutes, or until the lentils and vegetables are tender. Remove the bay leaf before serving.

Nutrition information per serving

Calories: 180; Carbs: 32g; Fat: 0.7g; Protein: 11g; Fiber: 15g

Low-Fat Minestrone with Cannellini Beans
VG, EG, DF, HF, GF, NF

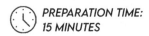 **PREPARATION TIME:** 15 MINUTES

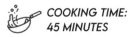 **COOKING TIME:** 45 MINUTES

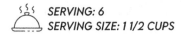 **SERVING: 6** SERVING SIZE: 1 1/2 CUPS

Ingredients

- 4 cups low-sodium vegetable broth
- 2 cups water
- 1 (14.5 oz) can low-sodium diced tomatoes
- 1 (15 oz) can cannellini beans, washed and strained
- 1 cup chopped carrots
- 1 cup chopped celery
- 1 cup chopped zucchini
- 1 cup chopped green bell pepper
- 1 cup chopped onion
- 2 cups chopped kale or spinach
- 3 cloves garlic, minced
- 2 tsp dried basil
- 2 tsp dried oregano
- 1 tsp dried thyme

Directions

1. Combine the vegetable broth, water, diced tomatoes, cannellini beans, carrots, celery, zucchini, bell pepper, onion, kale (or spinach), garlic, basil, oregano, and thyme in a large pot.
2. Bring the mixture to a boil over medium-high heat. Then, reduce the heat to medium-low and simmer for about 45 minutes, or until the vegetables are tender. Serve warm.

Nutrition information per serving
Calories: 155; Carbs: 28g; Fat: 0.7g; Protein: 9g; Fiber: 9g

SIDES & SNACKS

Sweet Potato Hummus | VG, EF, DF, HF, GF, NF

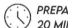 *PREPARATION TIME:*
20 MINUTES

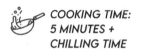 *COOKING TIME:*
5 MINUTES +
CHILLING TIME

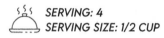 *SERVING: 4*
SERVING SIZE: 1/2 CUP

Ingredients

- 1 sweet potato, baked, skin removed
- 1 jar roasted red peppers, drained, blackened skin removed
- 3 tbsp lemon juice
- 1/2 tsp fresh garlic, finely diced
- 1/2 tsp ground cumin
- Pinch of cayenne pepper
- 1/4 tsp salt

Directions

1. Puree the sweet potato, roasted red peppers, lemon juice, garlic, cumin, cayenne, and salt in a food processor until smooth.
2. Transfer to a serving bowl and refrigerate for at least 1 hour to blend flavors.

Nutrition information per serving
Calories: 130; Carbs: 28g; Fat: 5g; Protein: 3g; Fiber: 3g

Grilled Fennel with Parmesan and Lemon

V, EF, GF, NF

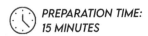 **PREPARATION TIME:**
15 MINUTES

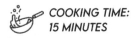 **COOKING TIME:**
15 MINUTES

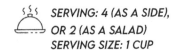 *SERVING: 4 (AS A SIDE),*
OR 2 (AS A SALAD)
SERVING SIZE: 1 CUP

Ingredients

- 3 Fennel bulbs, sliced for grilling
- Lemon juice, for drizzling
- Olive oil, for drizzling
- Shaved Parmesan (Parmigiano Reggiano)
- Salt and pepper, to taste

Directions

1. Preheat your grill or grill pan over medium-high heat.
2. Clean and slice the fennel bulbs into thick slices, ensuring they are suitable for grilling.
3. Drizzle the fennel slices with olive oil and season with salt and pepper.
4. Grill the fennel slices, turning once, until they are tender and have charred edges, about 5-7 minutes on each side.
5. Remove from the grill and immediately drizzle with lemon juice.
6. Finish by garnishing with shaved Parmesan cheese.

Nutrition information per serving

Calories: 58; Protein: 2g; Carbs: 7g; Fats: 3g; Fiber: 4g

Watermelon Feta Salad Bites | V, EF, GF, NF

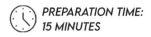 **PREPARATION TIME:** 15 MINUTES

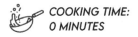 **COOKING TIME:** 0 MINUTES

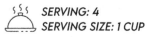 **SERVING:** 4
SERVING SIZE: 1 CUP

Ingredients

- 2 cups seedless watermelon, cubed
- 1/2 cup feta cheese, crumbled
- 1/4 cup fresh mint leaves, chopped
- 1/4 cup red onion, thinly sliced
- 1/4 cup cucumber, chopped
- Juice of half a lemon
- Black pepper, to taste

Directions

1. In a large bowl, gently mix the watermelon cubes, cucumber, and red onion.
2. Add the feta cheese and mint leaves. Toss gently to combine.
3. Squeeze lemon juice over the salad mixture and season with black pepper. Gently toss again to distribute the flavors.
4. Assemble the bites by piercing one each of the watermelon cubes, feta crumbles, and cucumber pieces onto toothpicks. Arrange them on a serving plate.
5. Drizzle any remaining dressing from the bowl over the assembled bites.

Nutrition information per serving

Calories: 88; Carbs: 11g; Fat: 3g; Protein: 4g; Fiber: 1g

Avocado Hummus with Veggies | VG, EF, DF, HF, GF, NF

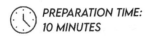 **PREPARATION TIME:** 10 MINUTES

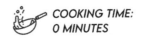 **COOKING TIME:** 0 MINUTES

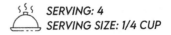 **SERVING: 4** SERVING SIZE: 1/4 CUP

Ingredients

- 1 ripe avocado, pitted and peeled
- 1 cup canned chickpeas, drained and rinsed
- 2 cloves garlic, minced
- 1/4 cup fresh lemon juice
- 2 tbsp tahini
- 1 tbsp extra virgin olive oil
- 1/4 tsp ground cumin
- Assorted raw veggies (carrot sticks, cucumber slices, cherry tomatoes, bell pepper strips) for dipping

Directions

1. In a food processor, combine the avocado, chickpeas, garlic, lemon juice, tahini, olive oil, and ground cumin. Blend until smooth.
2. Transfer the avocado hummus to a serving bowl.
3. Serve with an assortment of raw veggies for dipping.

Nutrition information per serving

Calories: 143; Carbs: 13g; Fat: 9g; Protein: 5g; Fiber: 6g

Smoked Salmon Pinwheels | EF, NF

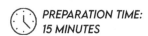 PREPARATION TIME:
15 MINUTES

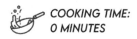 COOKING TIME:
0 MINUTES

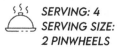 SERVING: 4
SERVING SIZE:
2 PINWHEELS

Ingredients

- 8 slices of smoked salmon
- 4 low-carb whole wheat tortillas
- 1 cup light cream cheese
- 1/2 cup thinly sliced cucumber
- 1/2 cup finely chopped dill
- Black pepper, to taste
- Lemon zest, for garnish

Directions

1. Spread light cream cheese evenly over each tortilla.
2. Place two slices of smoked salmon on top of the cream cheese on each tortilla.
3. Add cucumber slices and chopped dill over the salmon. Season with black pepper.
4. Roll up each tortilla tightly, wrap each roll in plastic wrap, and refrigerate for at least one hour to set.
5. After refrigeration, remove the plastic wrap and slice each roll into four pinwheels.
6. Arrange the pinwheels on a serving plate and garnish with lemon zest before serving.

Nutrition information per serving
Calories: 175; Carbs: 17g; Fat: 6g; Protein: 14g; Fiber: 3g

Spicy Roasted Chickpeas | VG, EF, DF, HF, GF, NF

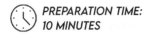 **PREPARATION TIME:**
10 MINUTES

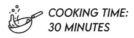 **COOKING TIME:**
30 MINUTES

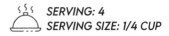 **SERVING: 4**
SERVING SIZE: 1/4 CUP

Ingredients

- 1 (15-oz) can chickpeas (low sodium), strained and washed
- 1 tbsp olive oil
- 1 tsp smoked paprika
- 1/2 tsp cayenne pepper
- 1/2 tsp garlic powder
- 1/4 tsp onion powder
- 1/2 tsp dried oregano
- Ground black pepper to taste

Directions

1. Preheat your oven to 400°F (200°C).
2. Lay the chickpeas on a clean kitchen towel to remove excess water.
3. In a large bowl, combine olive oil, smoked paprika, cayenne pepper, garlic powder, onion powder, dried oregano, and black pepper.
4. Add the chickpeas to the bowl and toss until they are evenly coated with the spice mixture.
5. Spread the chickpeas out on a parchment-lined baking sheet.
6. Bake for about 30 minutes, stirring occasionally, until crispy. Allow to cool down before serving.

Nutrition information per serving
Calories: 165; Carbs: 22g; Fat: 5g; Protein: 6g; Fiber: 6g

Baba Ghanoush | VG, EF, DF, GF, NF

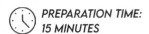 **PREPARATION TIME:**
15 MINUTES

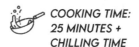 **COOKING TIME:**
25 MINUTES +
CHILLING TIME

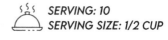 **SERVING: 10**
SERVING SIZE: 1/2 CUP

Ingredients

- 2 large eggplants (about 2 pounds)
- ½ cup tahini
- ½ cup fresh parsley, chopped
- 6 tbsp lemon juice
- 2 garlic cloves, crushed into a paste
- 1 tsp salt
- Pinch of cayenne pepper

Directions

1. Preheat the oven to 450° Fahrenheit. Place the eggplants on a baking sheet and prick them all over.
2. Bake for 25 minutes or until the skin is browned and the inside is soft.
3. After cooling, cut the eggplants in half lengthwise, drain off any excess liquid and loose seeds.
4. Scoop out the pulp and place it in a food processor.
5. Add the tahini, parsley, lemon juice, garlic, salt, and cayenne pepper. Blend until smooth and well mixed.
6. Garnish with additional chopped parsley and serve with 100% whole-grain pita or flatbread.

Nutrition information per serving
Calories: 100; Fat: 7g; Carbs: 9g; Protein: 3g; Fiber: 4g

Zesty Grilled Artichokes | VG, EF, DF, HF, GF, NF

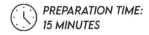 **PREPARATION TIME:**
15 MINUTES

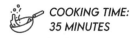 **COOKING TIME:**
35 MINUTES

SERVING: 4
SERVING SIZE:
1/4 OF THE RECIPE

Ingredients

- 2 large artichokes, halved and cleaned
- 1 lemon, juiced
- 1/4 cup rice vinegar
- 2 cloves garlic, minced
- 1/2 tsp dried oregano
- 1/4 tsp black pepper

Directions

1. Fill a large pot with water and add the lemon juice. Add the cleaned artichoke halves and bring to a boil. Cook for about 15 minutes until slightly tender.
2. In a small bowl, mix together the rice vinegar, minced garlic, dried oregano, and black pepper to create a zesty marinade.
3. Preheat the grill to medium heat.
4. Remove the boiled artichoke halves from the pot, allowing them to drain. Brush each artichoke half with the zesty marinade.
5. Place the marinated artichoke halves on the grill, cut side down. Grill for 8-10 minutes per side until charred.
6. Serve and enjoy the delicious char and zest on these grilled artichokes.

Nutrition information per serving
Calories: 60; Carbs: 11g; Fat: 0.5g; Protein: 3g; Fiber: 6g

Baked Sunchokes and Potatoes | VG, EF, DF, GF, NF

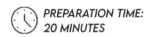 **PREPARATION TIME:**
20 MINUTES

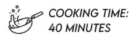 **COOKING TIME:**
40 MINUTES

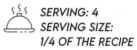 **SERVING: 4**
SERVING SIZE:
1/4 OF THE RECIPE

Ingredients

- 12 oz small to medium sunchokes
- 12 oz baby potatoes
- Kosher salt
- 2 tbsp. olive oil, divided
- 2 cloves garlic, finely chopped
- 2 tsp. smoked paprika
- 2 tsp. lemon juice
- Chopped parsley, for serving

Directions

1. In a large saucepan, combine the sunchokes and potatoes and cover with cold water. Bring to a boil. Reduce the heat and season with 2 tbsp of salt. Simmer until barely tender—7 to 8 minutes for potatoes, 11 to 13 minutes for sunchokes. Once done, transfer to a baking sheet.
2. Once the vegetables have cooled enough to handle, lightly crush them to break the skins. Heat 1 tbsp olive oil in a large skillet over medium-low heat. Cook the potatoes until golden brown and crisp, 3 to 4 minutes per side. Season with 1/4 tsp salt, then transfer to a plate. Continue with the remaining oil and sunchokes.
3. Sprinkle with paprika, toss with the vegetables, then mix in the lemon juice. Serve topped with parsley.

Nutrition information per serving
Calories: 152; Protein: 3g; Carbs: 25g; Fat: 5.5g; Fiber: 3g

Cucumber and Radish Slaw | VG, EF, DF, GF, NF

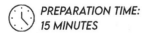 PREPARATION TIME:
15 MINUTES

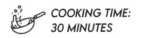 COOKING TIME:
30 MINUTES

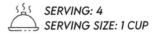 SERVING: 4
SERVING SIZE: 1 CUP

Ingredients

- 2 cups thinly sliced cucumber
- 1 cup thinly sliced radishes
- 1/4 cup chopped fresh parsley
- 1/4 cup chopped fresh cilantro
- 2 tbsp apple cider vinegar
- 2 tbsp fresh lemon juice
- 1 tbsp extra-virgin olive oil
- 1/4 tsp salt
- 1/8 tsp black pepper

Directions

1. In a large bowl, combine cucumber and radishes. Stir in chopped parsley and cilantro to mix well.
2. In a small bowl, whisk together apple cider vinegar, lemon juice, olive oil, salt, and black pepper.
3. Pour the dressing over the cucumber and radishes mixture, tossing to ensure an even coat.
4. Cover the slaw and refrigerate for at least 30 minutes before serving.

Nutrition information per serving
Calories: 60; Carbs: 4g; Fat: 4g; Protein: 1g; Fiber: 1g

Steamed Lemony Asparagus | VG, EF, DF, GF, NF

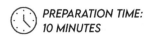 **PREPARATION TIME:**
10 MINUTES

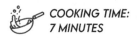 **COOKING TIME:**
7 MINUTES

SERVING: 4
SERVING SIZE:
5 ASPARAGUS SPEARS

Ingredients

- 20 asparagus spears, trimmed
- 1 lemon, zested and juiced
- 1 tbsp chopped fresh dill
- 1/2 tbsp extra-virgin olive oil

Directions

1. Fill your steamer with water and bring it to a boil. Place the asparagus in the steamer basket, and steam for about 5-7 minutes until they are tender-crisp.
2. In a small bowl, combine the lemon zest, lemon juice, chopped dill, and olive oil.
3. Once the asparagus is cooked, remove it from the steamer and gently toss with the lemon-dill mixture.
4. Serve immediately, offering a vibrant and flavorful side dish.

Nutrition information per serving
Calories: 35; Carbs: 4g; Fat: 2; Protein: 2g; Fiber: 2g

White Bean, Herb Dip with Crudites

VG, EF, DF, GF, NF

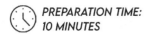 **PREPARATION TIME:**
10 MINUTES

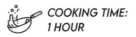 **COOKING TIME:**
1 HOUR

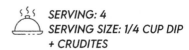 **SERVING: 4**
SERVING SIZE: 1/4 CUP DIP
+ CRUDITES

Ingredients

- 1 (15 oz) can of no-salt-added white beans, strained
- 2 tbsp fresh lemon juice
- 1 clove garlic, minced
- 2 tbsp chopped fresh parsley
- 1 tbsp chopped fresh chives
- 1 tbsp chopped fresh basil
- 1/4 tsp black pepper
- 1/4 cup water
- Assorted raw vegetables for dipping (carrots, cherry tomatoes, cucumber slices, bell pepper strips)

Directions

1. In a food processor, combine the white beans, lemon juice, garlic, parsley, chives, basil, and black pepper. Blend until smooth.
2. Gradually add water while blending to achieve your desired consistency for the dip.
3. Transfer the dip to a serving bowl and refrigerate for at least one hour to chill.
4. Serve the chilled white bean and herb dip with a variety of raw vegetables for dipping.

Nutrition information per serving

Calories: 146; Carbs: 21g; Fat: 1g; Protein: 10g; Fiber: 5g

SALADS

Cauliflower "Tabbouleh" | VG, EF, DF, HF, GF, NF

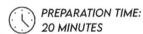 PREPARATION TIME:
20 MINUTES

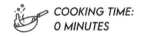 COOKING TIME:
0 MINUTES

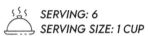 SERVING: 6
SERVING SIZE: 1 CUP

Ingredients

- 1 cauliflower
- 2 tomatoes
- 1 cucumber
- 180g pitted black olives
- Fresh mint leaves, to taste
- 2 tbsp olive oil
- Juice of 1/2 lemon

Directions

1. Cut the cauliflower into florets and place them in the blender. Pulse to achieve very small pieces (be careful not to overblend, as it may turn into a cream).
2. Transfer the cauliflower pieces to a bowl. Dice the tomatoes and cucumber, and mix them with the cauliflower. Then add the sliced black olives.
3. Wash and dry the mint leaves, chop them with scissors, and add them to the mixture.
4. Dress with olive oil and lemon juice, then mix well. Enjoy your meal!
5. Tip for optimal taste: For an enhanced flavor, it's recommended to let the tabbouleh rest in the refrigerator for about 30 minutes before serving.

Nutrition information per serving

Calories: 147; Carbs: 6g; Fat: 9g; Protein: 6g; Fiber: 8g

Italian Panzanella | VG, EF, DF, HF, NF

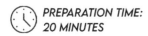 PREPARATION TIME: 20 MINUTES   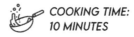 COOKING TIME: 10 MINUTES   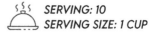 SERVING: 10 SERVING SIZE: 1 CUP

Ingredients

- 4 cups whole grain bread, cut into 1-inch cubes
- 3 tbsp red wine vinegar
- 1 tbsp white grape juice
- 1 tsp chia seed
- 1 tsp fresh garlic, finely minced
- 1/2 tsp dijon or whole grain mustard
- 3 tbsp extra virgin olive oil
- 1/2 tsp salt
- 1/2 tsp ground black pepper
- 5 cups ripe tomatoes (about 3 large), cut into 1-inch cubes
- 1 1/2 cups cucumber, unpeeled, seeded, sliced 1/2 inch
- 1/2 cup red onion, thinly sliced
- 3 cups arugula, firm packed
- 1 1/4 cups basil leaves (about 25), chiffonade

Directions

1. Preheat the oven to 350° F. Bake cubed whole grain bread on a nonstick baking sheet for 10 minutes, or until crisp and faintly coloured.
2. In a large mixing bowl, combine the vinegar, grape juice, chia seeds, garlic, mustard, olive oil, salt, and pepper. Set aside.
3. Remove the croutons from the oven and allow to cool. Combine the tomatoes, cucumber, and red onion with the vinaigrette and mix thoroughly. Then add the arugula, basil and croutons, stirring to combine.

Nutrition information per serving

Calories: 90; Fiber: 2g; Protein: 2g; Fat: 26g; Carbs: 9g

Mediterranean Tofu, Green Bean, and Olive Salad

VG, EF, DF, GF, NF

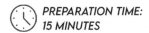 **PREPARATION TIME:** 15 MINUTES

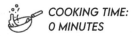 **COOKING TIME:** 0 MINUTES

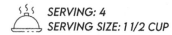 **SERVING:** 4 SERVING SIZE: 1 1/2 CUP

Ingredients

- 1 (14 oz) extra-firm tofu, drained & cubed
- 4 cups green beans, blanched & cooled
- 1 cup cherry tomatoes, halved
- 1/3 cup kalamata olives, pitted & halved
- 1/4 cup red onion, thinly sliced
- 1 medium cucumber, diced
- 2 tbsp freshly chopped parsley
- 2 tbsp fresh lemon juice
- 2 tbsp red wine vinegar
- 1 tbsp olive oil
- Salt & pepper, as required

Directions

1. In a large bowl, combine the cubed tofu, blanched green beans, cherry tomatoes, olives, red onion, and cucumber.
2. In a small bowl, whisk together lemon juice, vinegar, olive oil, salt, and pepper to create the dressing.
3. Drizzle the dressing over the tofu and vegetable mixture in the large bowl. Toss gently to ensure everything is well coated, then serve.

Nutrition information per serving

Calories: 190; Carbs: 17g; Fat: 9g; Protein: 13g; Fiber: 5g

Grilled Salmon & Spinach Salad | EF, DF, GF, NF

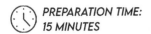 **PREPARATION TIME:**
15 MINUTES

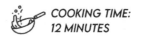 **COOKING TIME:**
12 MINUTES

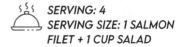 **SERVING: 4**
SERVING SIZE: 1 SALMON
FILET + 1 CUP SALAD

Ingredients

- 4 (4 oz each) salmon filets
- 8 cups baby spinach, washed and dried
- 1 cucumber, sliced thinly
- 2 cups cherry tomatoes, halved
- 1/2 small red onion, thinly sliced
- Juice of 1 lemon
- 2 tbsp extra-virgin olive oil
- Salt & pepper, as required

Directions

1. Preheat your grill over medium-high heat. Season the salmon filets with salt and pepper.
2. Grill the salmon filets for 6-7 minutes on each side, until fully cooked.
3. In a large salad bowl, combine the baby spinach, cucumber slices, cherry tomatoes, and red onion.
4. In a small bowl, whisk together lemon juice, olive oil, salt, and pepper to make a light vinaigrette.
5. Drizzle the vinaigrette over the salad and toss gently to combine.
6. Divide the salad among four plates and top each with a grilled salmon filet.

Nutrition information per serving

Calories: 318; Carbs: 8g; Fat: 18g; Protein: 32g; Fiber: 3g

Poached Shrimp, Bell Pepper, and Watercress Salad

EF, DF, GF, NF

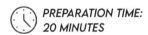 **PREPARATION TIME:** 20 MINUTES

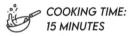 **COOKING TIME:** 15 MINUTES

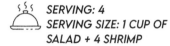 **SERVING: 4** SERVING SIZE: 1 CUP OF SALAD + 4 SHRIMP

Ingredients

- 16 large raw shrimp, peeled & deveined
- 4 cups watercress, washed and roughly chopped
- 2 medium bell peppers, deseeded & thinly sliced
- 1 medium cucumber, sliced into thin half-moons
- 1/4 cup rice vinegar
- 2 tsp honey
- Juice of one lemon
- Salt & pepper, to taste

Directions

1. In a large pot, bring water to a boil and season with salt. Add the shrimp and cook for 3 to 5 minutes until they are opaque. Transfer the shrimp to a plate and set aside to cool.
2. In a bowl, whisk together the rice vinegar, honey, lemon juice, salt, and pepper to create the dressing.
3. In a large salad bowl, combine the watercress, bell peppers, and cucumber. Drizzle the prepared dressing over the vegetables and gently toss to combine.
4. Add the cooled shrimp to the salad and toss again to distribute them evenly.
5. Serve the salad immediately.

Nutrition information per serving

Calories: 180; Carbs: 15g; Fat: 2g; Protein: 25g; Fiber: 3g

SPECIAL OCCASIONS RECIPES

Meat Mains

Roasted Chicken with Mediterranean Potatoes
DF, EF, GF, NF

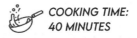 **PREPARATION TIME:** 25 MINUTES 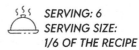 **COOKING TIME:** 40 MINUTES **SERVING:** 6 **SERVING SIZE:** 1/6 OF THE RECIPE

Ingredients
- 6 Chicken thighs
- 21 oz potatoes
- 3.5 oz cherry tomatoes
- 2.8 oz Taggiasca olives
- 1.4 oz capers
- 6 tbsp Cornmeal flour for breading
- 1 tsp Oregano
- 1 tsp Rosemary
- 1 Garlic cloves
- 1 onion
- Extra virgin olive oil
- Salt
- 5 Bay leaves

Directions
1. First, peel and chop the potatoes into pieces, then place them in a bowl full of water for about 20 minutes. Rinse several times to remove starch and then dry them.
2. In the meantime, season the chicken thighs with oil, salt, and pepper (and optional herbs). Let them rest for a few minutes, then ensure they are well coated in oil and dredge them in a bowl with cornmeal flour.
3. Prepare a baking dish, coat the bottom with a drizzle of oil, and arrange the potatoes around the sides. Add sliced onions and garlic on top, then the halved cherry tomatoes and season with salt. Add olives, capers, a handful of dried oregano, rosemary, and a few bay leaves.
4. Drizzle with olive oil and bake in a preheated oven at 190°C (374°F) for about 40 minutes. Then, remove from the oven and enjoy.

Nutrition information per serving
Calories: 450; Fat: 20g; Carbs: 35g; Protein: 25g; Fiber: 5g

Spaghetti & Meatballs | HF, NF

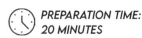 **PREPARATION TIME:** 20 MINUTES

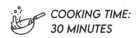 **COOKING TIME:** 30 MINUTES

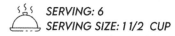 **SERVING: 6** SERVING SIZE: 1 1/2 CUP

Ingredients

- 1 large egg
- 3 tbsp finely chopped fresh basil (plus more for serving)
- 3 tbsp finely chopped fresh parsley
- 1 tsp dried oregano
- 3/4 tsp salt
- 1/4 tsp freshly ground black pepper
- 2 cloves garlic, minced
- 1/4 cup water
- 1 1/2 pounds ground "meatloaf mix" (equal parts ground beef, pork, and veal)
- 3/4 cup dried Italian-style bread crumbs
- 1/2 cup freshly grated Parmigiano-Reggiano cheese (plus more for serving)
- 1 large jar (32 oz) high-quality marinara sauce
- 1 pound spaghetti

Directions

1. Preheat your oven to 350°F. In a large mixing bowl, combine the eggs, basil, parsley, oregano, salt, pepper, garlic, and water.
2. Stir in the meat, breadcrumbs, and cheese until barely incorporated. Roll the mixture into golf-ball-sized meatballs and set them on an oiled baking sheet.
3. Bake for 10 minutes, then flip the meatballs and bake for another 10 minutes, or until browned and nearly cooked through.
4. In a large skillet, reduce the marinara sauce to a simmer. Adjust the seasoning to taste. Cover and simmer for 10 minutes.
5. Boil the pasta in well-salted water until "al dente". Drain and combine with sauce and meatballs. Garnish with fresh basil and additional grated cheese.

Nutrition information per serving

Calories: 731; Fat: 29g; Carbs: 78g; Sugar: 11g; Fiber: 6g

Moussaka

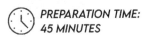 PREPARATION TIME: 45 MINUTES

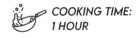 COOKING TIME: 1 HOUR

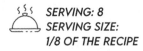 SERVING: 8
SERVING SIZE: 1/8 OF THE RECIPE

Ingredients

- 3 eggplants, peeled and cut lengthwise into 1/2 inch thick slices
- 1/4 cup olive oil
- 1 tbsp butter
- 1 pound lean ground beef
- 2 onions, chopped
- 1 clove garlic, minced
- Ground black pepper, to taste
- 2 tbsp dried parsley
- 1/2 tsp fines herbs
- 1/4 tsp ground cinnamon
- 1/2 tsp ground nutmeg, divided
- 1 can tomato sauce
- 1/2 cup red wine
- 1 egg, beaten
- 4 cups milk
- 1/2 cup butter
- 6 tbsp all-purpose flour
- Ground white pepper, to taste
- 1 1/2 cups freshly grated Parmesan cheese

Directions

1. Place eggplant slices on paper towels, sprinkle lightly with salt, and let aside for 30 minutes. Pat dry.
2. Fry eggplant in olive oil until browned, then drain on paper towels.
3. Melt 1 tbsp butter and sauté ground beef, onions, and garlic. Season. Combine the parsley, fine herbs, cinnamon, 1/4 tsp nutmeg, tomato sauce, and wine. Simmer for 20 minutes, then let cool before stirring in the egg.
4. Scald milk. Melt 1/2 cup butter; whisk in flour, then gradually add milk and whisk until thickened. Season with salt and white pepper.
5. Preheat the oven to 350°F (175°C). In a baking dish, combine eggplant, meat sauce, and Parmesan. Pour béchamel on top, then sprinkle with nutmeg and the remaining cheese.
6. Bake for approximately one hour, or until bubbling and golden.

Nutrition information per serving
Calories: 567; Fat: 39g; Carbs: 29g; Protein: 24g; Fiber: 2g

Fish Mains

Soy Ginger Salmon | EF, DF, GF, NF

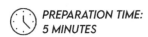 **PREPARATION TIME:**
5 MINUTES

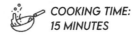 **COOKING TIME:**
15 MINUTES

SERVING: 2
SERVING SIZE:
1/2 OF THE RECIPE

Ingredients
- 3 tbsp low-sodium soy sauce
- 1 tbsp rice vinegar
- 2 cloves garlic, minced (about 2 tsp)
- 2 tsp grated fresh ginger
- 1 tsp honey
- 1/2 tsp garlic-chili paste, sriracha, or 1/4 tsp red pepper flakes
- 1 pound skin-on salmon filet, at room temperature, cut into 3-4 portions
- 2 tsp extra-virgin olive oil
- Chopped green onions, for serving
- Toasted sesame seeds, for serving

Directions
1. Preheat your oven to 425 degrees Fahrenheit and position a rack in the middle. Heat a large cast-iron pan or other robust, ovenproof skillet over high heat for at least 10 minutes, until extremely hot.
2. In a small saucepan, mix together the soy sauce, rice vinegar, garlic, and ginger. Bring to a simmer over medium-high heat, then remove and mix in the honey and chili paste. Reserve a few spoonfuls of the glaze for serving.
3. Drizzle the salmon with olive oil and brush it evenly. Place the salmon skin side up in a heated skillet. Cook, undisturbed, for about 3 minutes, or until crust develops.
4. Flip the salmon skin-side down, coat with the glaze, and immediately place the skillet in the oven. Bake for about 6 minutes, until the salmon is tender and flaky.
5. Allow the salmon to rest for 4 to 5 minutes after taking it from the oven, covered with foil.
6. Serve the salmon with the remaining glaze, sliced green onions, and sesame seeds.

Nutrition information per serving
Calories: 338; Carbs: 9g; Protein: 45g; Fat: 13g; Fiber: 1g

Mediterranean Seafood Gratin | EF, NF

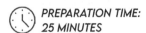 PREPARATION TIME:
25 MINUTES

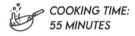 COOKING TIME:
55 MINUTES

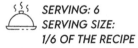 SERVING: 6
SERVING SIZE:
1/6 OF THE RECIPE

Ingredients

- 3 tbsp olive oil
- 1 large onion, thinly sliced
- 1 fennel bulb, trimmed and thinly sliced
- 3 large garlic cloves, finely sliced
- 1 heaped tsp coriander seeds, lightly crushed
- 5 tbsp white wine or vegetable stock
- 2 cans (28 oz) chopped tomatoes with herbs
- 2 tbsp tomato purée
- 1 bay leaf
- 1 tbsp fresh lemon juice
- 1 small bunch flat-leaf parsley, leaves roughly chopped
- 2 lb mixed skinless fish filets, cut into chunks
- 12 oz raw peeled king prawns
- 2.5 oz finely grated Parmesan
- 2 oz panko or coarse dried breadcrumbs

Directions

1. Preheat the oven to a moderate temperature.
2. Sauté Vegetables: In a large skillet, heat the olive oil over medium heat. Add the onion, fennel, and garlic, cooking until softened. Stir in the coriander seeds and cook for another minute.
3. Add Liquids: Pour in the white wine or vegetable stock, bringing it to a simmer. Add the chopped tomatoes, tomato purée, and bay leaf. Simmer for 15 minutes, allowing the flavors to meld.
4. Season: Stir in the lemon juice and half of the chopped parsley. Taste and adjust seasoning as necessary.
5. Prepare Seafood: Place the fish chunks and prawns in a large baking dish. Pour the tomato and vegetable mixture over the seafood, ensuring even coverage.
6. Topping: Mix the Parmesan with the breadcrumbs and sprinkle over the top of the gratin.
7. Bake: Place the dish in the preheated oven and bake for 40 minutes, or until the seafood is cooked through and the topping is golden and crispy.
8. Serve: Garnish with the remaining parsley and serve hot with a green salad on the side if desired.

Nutrition information per serving

Calories: 350; Carbs: 15g; Protein: 30g; Fat: 18g; Fiber: 3g

Steamed Lobster Tail with Mango Salsa | EF, DF, GF, NF

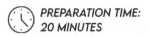 **PREPARATION TIME:**
20 MINUTES

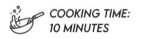 **COOKING TIME:**
10 MINUTES

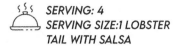 **SERVING: 4**
SERVING SIZE:1 LOBSTER
TAIL WITH SALSA

Ingredients

- 4 lobster tails (about 5 oz each)
- 1 ripe mango, peeled, pitted, and diced
- 1/2 small red onion, finely chopped
- 1/2 small red bell pepper, chopped
- Juice of 1 lime
- 2 tbsp chopped fresh cilantro
- Salt and pepper, to taste

Directions

1. Fill your large steamer with water and bring to a boil. Place the lobster tails in the steamer basket, cover, and steam for 7 to 8 minutes, or until the shells turn bright red.
2. While the lobster is steaming, prepare the mango salsa. In a medium bowl, combine the diced mango, chopped red onion, red bell pepper, lime juice, and chopped cilantro. Season the salsa with salt and pepper to taste. Mix well to ensure the flavors meld.
3. Once the lobster tails are done steaming, remove them from the steamer and let them cool for a few minutes until they are safe to handle. Carefully remove the lobster meat from the shells.
4. To serve, place each cooked lobster tail on a plate and generously top with the mango salsa.

Nutrition information per serving
Calories: 208; Carbs: 18g; Fat: 3g; Protein: 29g; Fiber: 2g

Seafood Paella | GF, NF

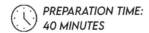 **PREPARATION TIME:**
40 MINUTES

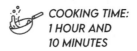 **COOKING TIME:**
1 HOUR AND
10 MINUTES

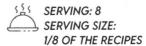 **SERVING: 8**
SERVING SIZE:
1/8 OF THE RECIPES

Ingredients

- 20-24 raw shell-on king prawns
- 2 tbsp olive oil
- 18 oz monkfish, cut into chunks
- 1 large onion, finely chopped
- 18 oz paella rice
- 4 garlic cloves, sliced
- 2 tsp smoked paprika
- 1 tsp cayenne pepper (optional)
- Pinch of saffron
- 2 cans (28 oz) chopped tomatoes (save the rest for the stock)
- 18 oz mussels, cleaned
- 3.5 oz frozen peas
- 3.5 oz frozen baby broad beans
- A handful of parsley leaves, roughly chopped

For the Stock:

- 2 litres of water
- 1 tbsp olive oil
- 1 onion, roughly chopped
- 1/2 can (7 oz) chopped tomatoes
- 6 garlic cloves, roughly chopped
- 1 vegetable stock cube
- 1 star anise

Directions

1. Peel and devein the prawns, keeping the heads and shells.
   Store the prawns in the refrigerator.
2. To make stock: Heat the oil in a big pan over medium-high
   heat. Combine the onion, tomatoes, garlic, and conserved
   prawn shells and heads. Cook for 3–4 minutes. Pour in 2 liters
   of water, then add the vegetable stock cube and star anise.
   Bring to a boil, then simmer for 30 minutes. Allow to cool
   somewhat, then mix in batches and pour through a fine sieve.

3. Brown the monkfish in a paella pan or large frying pan for a few minutes on each side before removing and setting aside. Add the onion to the pan and cook until tender.
4. Stir in the rice and toast for 30 seconds. Cook for an additional 30 seconds after adding the garlic, paprika, cayenne (if using), and saffron.
5. Combine the tomatoes and 1.5 liters of fish stock. Bring to a boil, then reduce to a simmer and cook for approximately 10 minutes, stirring occasionally. Restore the monkfish, prawns, mussels, peas, and broad beans.
6. Cover the pan with a large baking tray or foil and cook for another 10-15 minutes, or until the mussels open and the prawns are fully cooked. Sprinkle with parsley before serving.

Nutrition information per serving
Calories: 384; Carbs: 54g; Fat: 6g; Protein: 26g; Fiber: 5g

Vegetarian Mains

Veggie Lasagna | V, NF

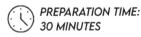 PREPARATION TIME:
30 MINUTES

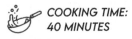 COOKING TIME:
40 MINUTES

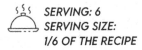 SERVING: 6
SERVING SIZE:
1/6 OF THE RECIPE

Ingredients

- 9 oz fresh lasagna sheets
- 4 cups of bechamel sauce
- 9 oz ricotta cheese
- 5 oz scamorza cheese, diced
- 2 large zucchinis, sliced into thin rounds
- 2 carrots, peeled and sliced into thin rounds
- 1 leek, thinly sliced
- 7 oz mushrooms (champignon), sliced
- 7 oz cherry tomatoes, cut into rounds
- Olive oil (extra virgin), as needed
- Salt and pepper, to taste

Directions

1. Begin by preparing the vegetables. Slice the zucchinis, carrots, leek, and mushrooms. Heat a drizzle of olive oil in a large skillet and start by sautéing the leeks, then add the carrots followed by the zucchinis, and finally the mushrooms.
2. Wash and slice the cherry tomatoes into rounds, then add them to the skillet with the other vegetables. Season with salt and pepper to taste.
3. Prepare 1 liter of bechamel sauce. Start by spreading a layer of bechamel in the bottom of a glass baking dish. Arrange a layer of lasagna sheets over the bechamel, then cover with the vegetable mixture, dollops of ricotta, and pieces of scamorza cheese. Cover with another generous layer of bechamel sauce.
4. Continue layering with lasagna sheets, vegetables, ricotta, scamorza cheese, and bechamel. Finish with a layer of lasagna sheets topped with bechamel sauce.
5. Preheat the oven to 356°F. Bake the lasagna for 40 minutes. Allow it to set for about ten minutes before serving.
6. Your Veggie Lasagna is now ready to be served. Enjoy this vegetarian feast that's sure to satisfy everyone at the table.

Nutrition information per serving

Calories: 400; Carbs: 45g; Fat: 18g; Protein: 18g; Fiber: 5g

Parmesan Hasselback Potatoes | V, EF, GF, NF

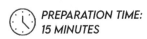 **PREPARATION TIME:** 15 MINUTES

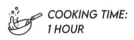 **COOKING TIME:** 1 HOUR

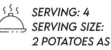 **SERVING:** 4
SERVING SIZE:
2 POTATOES AS A SIDE,
4 POTATOES AS A MAIN

Ingredients

- 4 large sweet potatoes
- 2 tbsp olive oil
- 1/2 cup grated Parmesan cheese
- 1/4 cup balsamic glaze
- Fresh herbs (such as thyme or rosemary), for garnish
- Salt and pepper, to taste

Directions

1. Preheat your oven to 425°F (220°C). Line a baking sheet with parchment paper.
2. Carefully slice each sweet potato crosswise at 1/8-inch intervals, being careful not to cut all the way through.
3. Place the sweet potatoes on the prepared baking sheet. Brush them with olive oil, ensuring it gets in between the slices. Season with salt and pepper.
4. Roast in the preheated oven for about 1 hour, or until the sweet potatoes are tender and the edges are crispy.
5. Remove from the oven and immediately drizzle with balsamic glaze, then sprinkle with grated Parmesan cheese.
6. Garnish with fresh herbs before serving. Enjoy warm as a delightful side or a savory main dish over baby greens.

Nutrition information per serving
Calories: 302; Carbs: 48g; Fat: 10g; Protein: 6g; Fiber: 4g

Aubergine Parmigiana | V, GF, NF

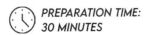 **PREPARATION TIME:**
30 MINUTES

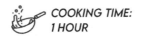 **COOKING TIME:**
1 HOUR

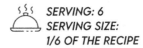 **SERVING: 6**
SERVING SIZE:
1/6 OF THE RECIPE

Ingredients

- 3 large firm aubergines, sliced 1cm thick
- Olive oil, for cooking
- 1 onion, finely chopped
- 1/2 bulb of spring garlic, or 1 clove of regular garlic, finely sliced
- 1 heaped tsp dried oregano
- 2 cans (28 oz) of quality plum tomatoes, or 1kg fresh ripe tomatoes
- A splash of wine vinegar
- 5 leaves of fresh basil
- 3 large handfuls of freshly grated Parmesan cheese
- 2 handfuls of dried breadcrumbs
- A few sprigs of fresh oregano, finely chopped
- 5 oz buffalo mozzarella (optional)

Directions

1. Preheat a griddle pan or barbecue. Lightly oil and grill the aubergine slices until lightly charred on both sides. Set aside.
2. In a pan over medium heat, sauté onion and garlic with dried oregano in olive oil until onion is soft and garlic is slightly colored.
3. For the sauce, if using tinned tomatoes, break them up. For fresh tomatoes, blanch, cool, peel, deseed, and chop. Add tomatoes to the onion mixture, cover, and simmer for 15 minutes until thickened.
4. Season the sauce with salt, pepper, and a splash of wine vinegar. Stir in torn basil leaves.
5. In a 15cm x 25cm baking dish, layer tomato sauce, a sprinkle of Parmesan, and grilled aubergine slices. Repeat, finishing with a layer of sauce and Parmesan.
6. Mix breadcrumbs with chopped fresh oregano and olive oil, and sprinkle over the top layer of Parmesan. Add torn mozzarella if using.
7. Bake at 190°C (375°F) for 30 minutes, or until golden and bubbly.
8. Serve hot and enjoy the melding of robust flavors and textures.

Nutrition information per serving

Calories: 237; Carbs: 15g; Fat: 14g; Protein: 14g; Fiber: 4g

DESSERTS

Grilled Peaches with Honey and Yogurt
V, EG, GF, NF

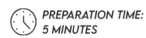 **PREPARATION TIME:** 5 MINUTES

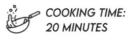 **COOKING TIME:** 20 MINUTES

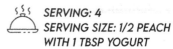 **SERVING: 4** SERVING SIZE: 1/2 PEACH WITH 1 TBSP YOGURT

Ingredients
- 1/4 cup fat-free vanilla Greek yogurt
- 1/8 tsp cinnamon
- 2 large ripe peaches, halved and pitted
- 2 tbsp honey, local and raw preferred

Directions
1. Prep the Yogurt Mixture: In a small bowl, mix together the fat-free vanilla Greek yogurt and cinnamon. Set aside for serving.
2. Preheat your grill to a low heat or set up for indirect grilling. Place peach halves on the grill, cut side down. Cover and grill until the peaches are soft, about 2 to 4 minutes per side. The goal is to achieve a slight char and warmth throughout the fruit without burning.
3. Once grilled to perfection, transfer the peach halves to serving plates. Drizzle each peach half with honey, then top with a tbsp of the prepared cinnamon yogurt.
4. Dive into this summery treat that perfectly balances the natural juiciness of peaches with the creamy tang of Greek yogurt and the sweet allure of honey.

Nutrition information per serving
Calories: 78; Carbs: 19g; Protein: 2g; Fat: 3g; Fiber: 2g

Roasted Pears in Orange Glaze| VG, EG, DF, HF, GF

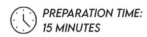 **PREPARATION TIME:**
15 MINUTES

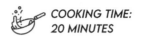 **COOKING TIME:**
20 MINUTES

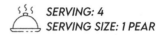 **SERVING: 4**
SERVING SIZE: 1 PEAR

Ingredients

- 4 small pears, peeled, halved, and cored
- 1/3 cup fresh orange juice
- 1/4 tsp orange zest
- 1/4 tsp cinnamon
- A pinch of nutmeg
- 2 tsp brown sugar

Directions

1. Start by preheating your oven to 350°F (175°C) to ensure it's ready for roasting the pears.
2. In a small bowl, whisk together the fresh orange juice, orange zest, cinnamon, nutmeg, and sugar until the mixture is well combined and the stevia has dissolved. This creates your flavorful orange glaze.
3. Place the pear halves in an oven-safe dish, cut side up. Ensure they are spaced out evenly to allow for uniform roasting.
4. Drizzle the prepared orange glaze evenly over the pear halves, making sure each piece is nicely coated with the mixture for maximum flavor.
5. Bake the pears in the preheated oven for about 20 minutes, or until they are tender when pierced with a fork. The exact time may vary depending on the size and ripeness of the pears.
6. Once tender and beautifully roasted, remove the pears from the oven. Serve them warm as a delightful dessert or a special treat. They can be enjoyed as is or paired with a scoop of vanilla ice cream or a dollop of whipped cream.
7.

Nutrition information per serving

Calories: 98; Carbs: 24g; Protein: 1g; Fat: 0g; Fiber: 5g

Vanilla Bean Panna Cotta | V, EF, GF

 PREPARATION TIME: 15 MINUTES

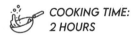 **COOKING TIME:** 2 HOURS

 SERVING: 4 SERVING SIZE: 1/4 CUP

Ingredients

- 1 envelope of unflavored gelatin (about 2 1/2 tsp)
- 3/4 cup unsweetened almond milk, divided
- 3/4 cup nonfat Greek yogurt
- 1/3 cup sugar
- 1 vanilla bean, split & seeds scraped

Directions

1. Gelatin Preparation: In a small bowl, sprinkle the gelatin over 1/4 cup of almond milk. Allow it to stand for 5 minutes until the gelatin has softened, absorbing the liquid.
2. In a saucepan, combine the remaining 1/2 cup of almond milk, nonfat Greek yogurt, sugar, and the scraped seeds from the vanilla bean. This mixture will infuse the panna cotta with a deep vanilla flavor.
3. Warm the mixture over medium-low heat, stirring often to ensure the ingredients are well combined and the sugar dissolves. Heat until the mixture is warm but not boiling, to preserve the delicate texture of the yogurt.
4. Remove the saucepan from the heat, then whisk in the softened gelatin until it is completely dissolved into the mixture, ensuring a smooth consistency.
5. Pour the mixture through a sieve into a large bowl to remove any lumps or remaining bits of gelatin, ensuring a perfectly smooth panna cotta.
6. Evenly divide the mixture among four small ramekins. Refrigerate for at least two hours, or until the panna cotta is fully set and chilled.
7. Once set, serve the Vanilla Bean Panna Cotta as a sophisticated and refreshing dessert. It can be garnished with fresh berries, mint, or a drizzle of honey for an extra touch of elegance.

Nutrition information per serving

Calories: 75; Carbs: 5g; Fat: 8g; Protein: 6g; Fiber: 2g

No-Bake Dark Chocolate Walnut Dessert Bars
VG, EF, DF, GF

 PREPARATION TIME:
15 MINUTES

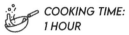 **COOKING TIME:**
1 HOUR

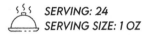 **SERVING: 24**
SERVING SIZE: 1 OZ

Ingredients

- 1 cup toasted walnuts
- 1½ cups golden raisins
- 5 brown rice cakes
- ¼ tsp cinnamon
- 1 tbsp vanilla extract
- 2 tbsp orange juice
- 5 oz of 70% dark bittersweet chocolate
- 5 tbsp orange juice or unsweetened alternative milk (soy, almond, etc.)
- 1 tbsp instant coffee (optional)

Directions

1. Prepare Walnut Mixture: In a food processor, pulse the toasted walnuts until they are finely ground. Add the golden raisins and pulse again until the mixture becomes sticky.
2. Incorporate the brown rice cakes and pulse until the mixture is fine and loose. Add cinnamon, vanilla extract, and 2 tbsp of orange juice, processing until the mixture reaches a gummy/sticky consistency.
3. Transfer the mixture to an 8"x 8" glass baking dish, spreading it evenly. Cover with plastic wrap and use a flat-bottomed object to press down firmly, ensuring the mixture is evenly distributed across the pan. Remove the plastic wrap afterward.
4. Prepare Chocolate Topping: In a double boiler over low heat, combine the dark chocolate, 5 tbsp of orange juice (or unsweetened alternative milk), and instant coffee if using. Stir continuously until the chocolate is fully melted and the mixture is smooth.
5. Pour the melted chocolate mixture over the pressed walnut base. Cover and refrigerate for at least one hour, or until the chocolate is set.
6. Cut into 24 portions and enjoy

Nutrition information per serving
Calories: 100; Carbs: 13g; Fat:13g; Protein: 2g; Fiber: 2g

Italian Tiramisu | V, EF, NF

 PREPARATION TIME:
30 MINUTES

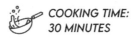 **COOKING TIME:**
30 MINUTES

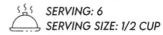 **SERVING: 6**
SERVING SIZE: 1/2 CUP

Ingredients

- 1 cup double cream
- 1 cup mascarpone cheese
- 1/3 cup Marsala wine
- 5 tbsp golden caster sugar
- 1 1/4 cups coffee, brewed from 2 tbsp coffee granules and 1 1/4 cups boiling water
- 1 3/4 cups sponge fingers
- 1 oz dark chocolate
- 2 tsp cocoa powder

Directions

1. In a large bowl, mix the double cream, mascarpone cheese, Marsala wine, and golden caster sugar. Whisk until the mixture is thoroughly combined and has reached the consistency of thickly whipped cream.
2. Pour the brewed coffee into a shallow dish. Dip a few sponge fingers at a time into the coffee, turning them for a few seconds until they are nicely soaked but not soggy.
3. In your chosen dish, create a layer using half of the soaked sponge fingers. Over this, spread half of the creamy mascarpone mixture.
4. Grate most of the dark chocolate over the first layer using the coarse side of a grater.
5. Repeat the process with the remaining sponge fingers and mascarpone mixture, finishing with a layer of the cream mixture.
6. Cover the dish and chill in the refrigerator for a few hours or preferably overnight. This tiramisu can be kept in the fridge for up to two days.
7. Before serving, dust the top with cocoa powder and grate the remaining dark chocolate over the top for a beautifully finished look.

Nutrition information per serving

Calories: 853; Fat: 73g; Carbs: 44g; Protein: 5g; Fiber: 2g

Meal Plan

The Importance of a Weekly Menu

The hustle and bustle of everyday life inevitably leads us to sideline the "what to cook for dinner" question, so often we arrive tired or at the last minute ending up preparing something quick, if not even opening the fridge and choosing the simplest, tastiest, and quickest solution... in these cases, the choice hardly reflects the balanced and healthy meal that the Mediterranean diet suggests and, in the long run, this behavior leads to a drift with serious repercussions on our health and that of the people living with us.

A weekly menu helps eliminate the torment of "What should I cook?" and allows you to stay in full control of your diet, enabling you to achieve the health goals you've set for yourself.

What Is a Weekly Menu?

Following a meal plan means planning the week's meals in advance, starting with what you put in the cart when you go shopping. If your goal is also weight loss, planning breakfast and snacks is a good habit because it reduces the margin of variability and trains your body, and your mind, to adhere to new standards.

Why Plan a Weekly Menu?

The reasons are various but mainly with a meal plan you can:

1. Optimize time and improve health: meal planning could be a potential tool to compensate for the lack of time and thus encourage meal preparation at home. This habit has been linked to a better diet quality and avoids the stress of having to repeatedly think and decide what to eat, with the risk of making wrong choices. Plus, having a guideline, many preparations can be anticipated the day before, limiting yourself to just assembling the dish.

2. Vary the diet: the difficulty of organizing with shopping and meal preparation carries the risk of always eating the same things. Planning helps, on the one hand, to not get bored of the diet and, on the other, to adhere to it

in the deepest possible way: the one that also embraces the nutritional variety linked to seasonality and the synergistic complementarity of various foods.

      3. Reduce waste and therefore make your wallet happy. Planning and preparing a careful shopping list that reflects the weekly menu helps you not to succumb to the temptation of buying "wrong foods," but also to consume everything that is bought. There's another strategy to make our wallet smile: taking advantage of turning on the oven to cook more foods for various meals or cooking more cereals at once for more meals that can be stored in the refrigerator for 3-4 days, seasoning them in different ways. Moreover, knowing the seasonality of foods, you can try to reduce the cost of fruits and vegetables.

28-Day Meal Plan to Achieve Health and Wellness

Week 1

Day 1

Breakfast	Coffee or tea with a bowl of Orange-Spiced Overnight Oats	p.58
Snack	Handful of almonds or walnuts	
Lunch	Chicken-Vegetable Quinoa Stew	p.98
Snack	Apple with nut butter	
Dinner	Bean and Spinach Rice Casserole	p.82

Day 2

Breakfast	Coffee or tea with Greek Yogurt Berry Parfait	p.64
Snack	Spicy Roasted Chickpeas	p.108
Lunch	Leftover Bean and Spinach Rice Casserole of Day 1 - Week 1	p.82
Snack	A peach (or apple, depending on the season)	
Dinner	Broccoli & Chicken Rice Skillet	p.88

Day 3

Breakfast	Green Smoothie Bowl with Berries	p.72
Snack	1/4 avocado mashed with lemon juice and salt on top of whole-grain crackers	
Lunch	Triple Mushroom Barley Soup	p.99
Snack	Package of olives and fresh veggies	
Dinner	Creamy Spinach-Artichoke Salmon served with bulgur wheat	p.75

Day 4

Breakfast	Coffee or tea Seasonal Fruit Breakfast Bowl	p.60
Snack	Pistachios	
Lunch	Whole Wheat Spaghetti with Vegetable Pesto	p.93
Snack	Greek yogurt with fresh fruit	
Dinner	Marinated Broiled Tuna Steaks with bulgur wheat and a tomato salad	p.79

Day 5

Breakfast	Coffee or tea and Peach & Raspberry Greek Yogurt Bowl	p.59
Snack	Dried apricots and walnuts	
Lunch	Mediterranean Tofu, Green Bean, and Olive Salad with a slice of whole-grain bread	p.117
Snack	Whole-grain crackers and black bean dip	
Dinner	Italian Baked Shrimp with Zucchini Spaghetti	p.77

Day 6

Breakfast	Coffee or tea and Cottage Cheese and Tomato Toast	p.71
Snack	In-season fruit (such as a peach or two apricots in summer, or a pear in winter)	
Lunch	Stuffed Eggplants with Rice	p.80
Snack	Piece of cheese and olives	
Dinner	Rosemary Garlic Lamb Loin Chops with couscous	p.92

Day 7

Breakfast	Coffee or tea with a bowl of Orange-Spiced Overnight Oats	p.58
Snack	Sliced orange and pistachios	
Lunch	A piece of whole-grain bread with Zesty Grilled Artichokes	p.110
Snack	Packaged, flavored lupini beans	
Dinner	Hearty Lentil and Vegetable Soup	p.101

Week 2

Day 1

Breakfast	Coffee or tea and Broccoli & Swiss Cheese Egg Cups	p.69
Snack	Spicy Roasted chickpeas	p.108
Lunch	Prosciutto, Mozzarella, and Melon Salad	p.91
Snack	Mixed nuts with a piece of dark chocolate	
Dinner	Leftover Rosemary Garlic Lamb Loin Chops with couscous of Day 6 - Week 1	p.92

Day 2

Breakfast	Strawberries Banana Smoothie Delight	p.65
Snack	Mini peppers stuffed with hummus	
Lunch	Tuna Croquettes with Dill and Lemon served on a bed of spinach and whole-grain crackers	p.74
Snack	Piece of cheese with a piece of fruit	
Dinner	Low-Fat Minestrone with Cannellini Beans with whole-grain bread	p.102

Day 3

Breakfast	Coffee or tea and a bowl of Quinoa Porridge with Banana and Walnuts	p.61
Snack	Greek yogurt and a piece of fruit	
Lunch	Leftover Low-Fat Minestrone with Cannellini Beans with whole-grain bread of Day 2 - Week 2	p.102
Snack	Hummus with sliced raw veggies like red peppers, celery, and cucumber	
Dinner	Honey-Ginger Grilled Sardines with salad and couscous	p.76

Day 4

Breakfast	Coffee or tea and Leftover Broccoli & Swiss Cheese Egg Cups of Day 01 - Week 2	p.69
Snack	Apple with nut butter	
Lunch	Grilled Veggie & White Bean Whole Wheat Wrap	p.81
Snack	Greek yogurt dip with sliced veggies	
Dinner	Garlic and Lime Baked Grouper with Baked Sunchokes and Potatoes	p.78 p.111

Day 5

Breakfast	Coffee or tea and a small bowl of Chia Pudding with Fresh Fruit	p.62
Snack	Handful of lightly salted nuts (hazelnuts, pistachios, almonds, or a mix)	
Lunch	Light Italian Carbonara	p.94
Snack	Fruit salad	
Dinner	Leftover Garlic and Lime Baked Grouper with Baked Sunchokes and Potatoes of Day 4 - Week 2	p.78 p.111

Day 6

Breakfast	Coffee or tea and Cottage Cheese and Tomato Toast	p.71
Snack	Container of Greek yogurt	
Lunch	Grilled Salmon & Spinach Salad with whole-grain bread	p.118
Snack	Smashed avocado on whole-grain crackers	
Dinner	Baked Zucchini Parmesan Casserole with feta and served over polenta	p.85

Day 7

Breakfast	Coffee or tea and Yogurt with Bananas and Almond-Buckwheat Groats	p.63
Snack	Dried cranberries and mixed nuts	
Lunch	Whole Wheat Linguine with Mushroom Ragu	p.96
Snack	Olives and a few pita chips dipped in hummus	
Dinner	Eggplant Rollatini with Ricotta and Cucumber and Radish Slaw	p.86 p.112

Week 3

Day 1

Breakfast	Coffee or tea with a bowl of Tropical Fruit Yogurt Delight	p.66
Snack	Handful of almonds or walnuts	
Lunch	Tempeh Ratatouille on Whole Grain Rice and a cup of lentil soup	p.84
Snack	Sliced carrots, bell peppers, and cucumbers dipped in hummus	
Dinner	Creamy Sun-Dried Tomato and Shallot Chicken	p.89

Day 2

Breakfast	Strawberries Banana Smoothie Delight	
Snack	Spicy Roasted chickpeas	p.108
Lunch	Leftover Creamy Sun-Dried Tomato and Shallot Chicken of Day 1 - Week 3	p.89
Snack	A peach (or apple, depending on the season)	
Dinner	Baked Turkey & Spinach Meatballs and a side salad	p.87

Day 3

Breakfast	Coffee or tea with plain Greek yogurt topped with a drizzle of honey and walnuts	
Snack	1/4 avocado mashed with lemon juice and salt on top of whole-grain crackers	
Lunch	Creamy Mushroom Pasta	p.97
Snack	Package of olives and fresh veggies	
Dinner	Smoked Salmon Pinwheels with with a slice of whole-grain bread	p.107

Day 4

Breakfast	Coffee or tea and toasted whole-grain bread, sliced cheese, and strawberries	
Snack	Pistachios	
Lunch	Cauliflower, Fennel, and Leek Chowder with polenta	p.100
Snack	Greek yogurt with fresh fruit	
Dinner	Leftover Smoked Salmon Pinwheels with with a slice of whole-grain bread of Day 3 - Week 3	p.107

Day 5

Breakfast	Coffee or tea and Peach and Raspberry Greek Yogurt Bowl	p.59
Snack	Dried apricots and walnuts	
Lunch	Stuffed Eggplants with Rice	p.80
Snack	Whole-grain crackers and black bean dip	
Dinner	Italian Chicken & Veggie Casserole with bulgur wheat	p.90

Day 6

Breakfast	Coffee or tea and Almond Flour Berry Pancakes	p.67
Snack	In-season fruit (such as a peach or two apricots in summer, or a pear in winter)	
Lunch	Whole Wheat Linguine with Mushroom Ragu	p.96
Snack	Piece of cheese and olives	
Dinner	Rosemary Garlic Lamb Loin Chops with couscous	p.92

Day 7

Breakfast	Coffee or tea and Greek Yogurt Berry Parfait	p.64
Snack	Sliced orange and pistachios	
Lunch	A piece of whole-grain bread with Baked Tofu in Parchment	p.83
Snack	Packaged, flavored lupini beans	
Dinner	Hearty Lentil and Vegetable Soup	p.101

Week 4

Day 1

Breakfast	Coffee or tea and Seasonal Fruit Breakfast Bowl	p.60
Snack	Spicy Roasted chickpeas	p.108
Lunch	Leftover Rosemary Garlic Lamb Loin Chops with couscous of Day 6 - Week 3	p.92
Snack	Mixed nuts with a piece of dark chocolate	
Dinner	Citrus-Poached Sole filet, roasted potatoes, and zucchini	p.73

Day 2

Breakfast	Green Smoothie Bowl with Berries	p.72
Snack	Mini peppers stuffed with hummus	
Lunch	Poached Shrimp, Bell Pepper, and Watercress Salad and whole-grain crackers	p.112
Snack	Piece of cheese with a piece of fruit	
Dinner	Triple Mushroom Barley Soup	p.99

Day 3

Breakfast	Coffee or tea and Broccoli & Swiss Cheese Egg Cups	p.69
Snack	Greek yogurt and a piece of fruit	
Lunch	Leftover Triple Mushroom Barley Soup of Day 2 - Week 4	p.99
Snack	Hummus with sliced raw veggies like red peppers, celery, and cucumber	
Dinner	Creamy Sun-Dried Tomato and Shallot Chicken with couscous	p.89

Day 4

Breakfast	Coffee or tea and a slice of veggie frittata with avocado	
Snack	Apple with nut butter	
Lunch	Eggplant Rollatini with Ricotta and whole-grain bread	p.86
Snack	Greek yogurt dip with sliced veggies	
Dinner	Creamy Spinach-Artichoke Salmon with bulgur	p.75

Day 5

Breakfast	Coffee or tea and a small bowl of Yogurt with Bananas and Almond-Buckwheat Groats	p.63
Snack	Handful of lightly salted nuts (hazelnuts, pistachios, almonds, or a mix)	
Lunch	Light Italian Carbonara	p.94
Snack	Fruit salad	
Dinner	Leftover Creamy Spinach-Artichoke Salmon with bulgur of Day 4 - Week 4	p.75

Day 6

Breakfast	Coffee or tea and oatmeal with nut butter and blueberries	
Snack	Container of Greek yogurt	
Lunch	Chicken-Vegetable Quinoa Stew	p.98
Snack	Smashed avocado on whole-grain crackers	
Dinner	Grilled Fennel with Parmesan and Lemon with an egg and a slice of whole grain bread	p.104

Day 7

Breakfast	Coffee or tea and Almond Flour Berry Pancakes	p.67
Snack	Dried cranberries and mixed nuts	
Lunch	Leftover Chicken-Vegetable Quinoa Stew of Day 6 - Week 4	p.98
Snack	Olives and a few pita chips dipped in hummus	
Dinner	Steamed Lemony Asparagus with breadcrumbs and Parmesan	p.113

Behind the Diet

Living Like a Mediterranean

Living like a Mediterranean embodies the essence of enjoying food, celebrating joy, being healthy, and feeling good. Everything you've discovered in this book has already shown you that the Mediterranean diet is not just a dietary regimen but a true lifestyle. Living like a Mediterranean, embracing this way of life, means not only carefully selecting what ends up on the plate but adopting an entire life philosophy that celebrates the pleasure of the table, the importance of social bonds, the value of physical activity, and a deep respect for nature.

This more holistic Mediterranean vision, closer to the real values of tradition, promotes physical health and at the same time emotional and social well-being, highlighting how the quality of life derives not only from what we eat but also from how we live.

In the Mediterranean, meals are more than mere occasions for nourishment; they are sacred moments dedicated to sharing and celebrating life. The conviviality of Mediterranean meals, where families and friends gather to enjoy food together, strengthens social bonds and contributes to emotional well-being. This approach to food and life emphasizes the importance of how we eat, promoting mindful and unhurried food consumption, valuing every bite and every moment spent in good company.

Respect for nature is another pillar of the Mediterranean lifestyle. The focus on the seasonality of products, preference for local foods, and sustainability of farming practices are expressions of a deep connection with the land, a relationship with the environment that not only guarantees access to fresh and nutritious foods but also teaches the value of balance and harmony with the natural world.

Adopting a Mediterranean lifestyle, teaching it to one's children or grandchildren, means celebrating the joy of living, encouraging each of us to find a personal balance that nourishes the body, mind, and spirit. A commitment also aimed at future generations.

Move Like a Mediterranean

The concept of the Mediterranean lifestyle, in addition to highlighting the importance of a balanced diet, places a strong emphasis on physical activity, integrated as a natural part of everyday life. This approach doesn't necessarily require structured or daily sports exercise, but rather encourages regular movement through enjoyable activities like walking, swimming, or cycling. Integrating these habits not only improves physical health but also mental health, facilitating moments of relaxation and connection with the surrounding environment.

The modern challenge of sedentary lifestyle indeed requires a commitment and particular attention to reducing periods of inactivity, seizing every possible opportunity to move. Physical activity, as simple as a daily 30-minute walk, is the fundamental basis for overall well-being, which should then be complemented with other forms of daily movement to counteract the negative effects of a sedentary lifestyle.

To promote a structured approach to physical activity, the concept of the "physical activity pyramid" has been proposed, a visual guide illustrating the variety and amount of exercise recommended for maintaining optimal health. At the base of this pyramid, we find basic and accessible activities like brisk walking, suggested for at least 30 minutes a day. This represents the foundation on which to build an active lifestyle, enriched by more specific activities like aerobic exercises, stretching, and muscle strengthening, recommended 2-3 times a week.

Determining "how much" physical activity is necessary isn't straightforward because the right amount can vary significantly among individuals, complicating the definition of a universal standard. However, the World Health Organization has attempted to establish basic guidelines, differentiated by age groups.

- For children and adolescents aged 5 to 17 years, it's recommended to engage in at least one hour per day of moderate- to vigorous-intensity activity, supplemented with strength exercises, at least three times a week.

- Adults aged 18 to 64 years should aim for 150 minutes of moderate activity per week, or 75 minutes of more intense activity, with the addition of muscle-strengthening exercises at least twice a week.

- For seniors over 65-years-old, the recommendations are similar to those for adults, with particular attention to activities that improve balance to prevent falls.

These guidelines not only promote the active adoption of the Mediterranean lifestyle but also highlight the importance of personalizing physical activity based on individual needs, contributing to a happier and less sedentary society.

But why is physical activity of such crucial importance? Scientific research has extensively demonstrated its benefits: from increased cardiovascular efficiency and the capacity to manage physical effort, to the strengthening of the immune system, resulting in a lower frequency of illness among those who regularly engage in sports. Physical activity effectively combats overweight and obesity, regulates cholesterol, improves musculoskeletal efficiency offering aesthetic benefits, and provides psychological advantages, acting as an anti-stressor and improving willpower, self-confidence, and self-esteem. For children and adolescents, participating in movement games and other physical activities is essential for healthy physical development and represents a valuable tool for socialization. Sports and physical exercise also help prevent risk behaviors such as smoking, alcohol abuse, and drug use.

These reflections underscore the importance of adopting an active approach that includes a holistic view of health, promoting regular and personalized physical activity to improve the quality of life at all ages.

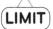

Physical Activity Pyramid

LIMIT

Limit physical inactivity and sedentary habits

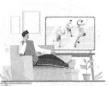

2-3 TIMES A WEEK

Partecipate in activities that increase flexibility, strength and endurance of the muscle

- Streching
- Sit and reach exercise
- Push Up
- Leg press

5-6 TIMES A WEEK

Accumulate al least 30 minutes per day of moderate intensity physical activity

- Brisk walking
- Cycling
- Swimming
- Aerobic exercise
- Dancing
- Skipping rope
- Basket ball
- Tennis
- Hiking

EVERYDAY

Accumulate al least 30 minutes per day of moderate intensity physical activity

- Walk up the stairs
- Walk to the shop
- Housework
- Gardening
- Walk to the office
- Park your car a distance away
- Increase walking each day
- Increase walking up and down stairs

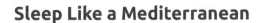

Sleep Like a Mediterranean

The Mediterranean diet and lifestyle also emerge as faithful allies of sleep, intertwining nutrition and well-being in an indissoluble bond. In this model, sleep is also a crucial element, powerfully anti-inflammatory, for a healthy and long life, and is closely tied to the choice and timing of our foods. Nutrients such as proteins, carbohydrates, and vitamins play a decisive role, thanks to their ability to regulate biological rhythms and promote the production of essential hormones like melatonin and serotonin. In particular, the intake of tryptophan, supported by vitamin B6 found in foods like bananas, is fundamental for the synthesis of these hormones and can significantly improve sleep quality. Cherries, peaches, and apricots prove to be valuable allies of the night, thanks to their content of magnesium, potassium, and tryptophan. Oats, with their supply of magnesium and calcium, also play a key role in promoting deep sleep.

Building a healthy Mediterranean dietary routine, constructing a good sleep-wake rhythm is another fundamental piece in combating chronic diseases, obesity, and dysfunctions.

Sleep duration shorter than recommendations is, in fact, correlated with more than double the risk of overweight and obesity due to neuroendocrine alterations, which change calorie intake, and metabolic alterations involving insulin sensitivity and glycemic homeostasis.

Following a Mediterranean style that promotes sleep also means limiting the evening consumption of junk food, alcohol, caffeine, and overly salty or spicy foods, which notoriously disturb proper rest and negatively impact well-being. The ideal Mediterranean dinner is consumed sitting at the table, at least three hours before lying down, should be light and balanced, favoring whole grains, vegetables, and light protein sources like fish and legumes, avoiding saturated fats and refined carbohydrates.

Not just nighttime rest, the Mediterranean model invites to rediscover in general the value of slowness and, when possible, the afternoon rest, a rural habit that in the Mediterranean basin some people, especially those who perform physical jobs, still maintain as a beneficial custom. In general, all specialists invite to take care of one's rest and to consider the quality of one's sleep as a fundamental indicator of overall health.

The Healthiest People's Habits

The secret to longevity, as we've seen, is the result of a balance between the health of the body and that of the mind, something that approaches the concept of happiness and well-being for humans. Therefore, to conclude this chapter, it seems useful to share the results of significant research on the habits adopted by the world's healthiest people. Many findings are evident and have been elaborated on in previous chapters, while others might seem unreachable when faced with the average lifestyle in our society. However, creating an ideal image of well-being to strive for and move towards is the first step toward the possibility of achieving or making a change in one's life if that's what you're looking for.

Here are the ten habits of the world's healthiest people:

1. Move More: Walking is the main mode of transport in the healthiest countries in the world. Daily moderate activity brings the most benefits and can be better for your body than high-intensity exercise. Good examples include gardening, playing with children, and walking the dog.

2. Know Your Purpose: Having a meaningful reason to get out of bed can help reduce stress and prevent diseases. Studies show that people who retire early often see a decline in their health and higher mortality rates compared to those who work.

3. De-stress: People living in healthy countries report less stress or know and practice techniques to alleviate it, such as meditation, breathing exercises, and somatic exercises.

4. Slow Down: Prioritize sleep, take vacations, or simply spend more time outdoors. Listen to your body and try not to push it to its limit but peacefully agree with its needs by allowing yourself to slow down and recover energy without ever fully depleting it.

5. Schedule Quiet Times: Activities like meditation and reading are great. Relaxing with a hot bath or dedicating time to hobbies that slow down thoughts and allow calming the mind should be part of your daily planning, like little rituals of happiness and self-care.

6. Follow the 80% Rule at Meals: Stop eating when you're 80% full. Wait ten minutes, then reevaluate your hunger. This rule prevents overeating, increases the mind-body connection, and promotes intentional and mindful eating.

7. Choose Natural Foods: People in healthy countries eat less processed food and more local, fresh, and natural food, as taught by the Mediterranean diet. Limit processed foods, sweets, and unnatural fats like margarine. Prepare as much food as possible from fresh and local sources. Knowing, as far as possible, the origin of what you eat is an exceptional way to deeply connect with what nourishes you.

8. Drink Plenty of Water and Herbal Tea, Avoid Soft Drinks: Herbal teas act as diuretics, lower blood pressure, and prevent heart disease.

9. Belong to a Healthy Social Network: A strong and supportive social system is crucial for reducing stress and living a healthy life. There is a strong biological link between social connection and our body's functioning. In 1995, the average American had three close friends—that number has dropped to two. Raising the average again is within your reach, and you can consider it a personal responsibility.

10. Focus on Face-to-Face Interactions Instead of Online to Improve Your Health and Happiness: The internet and technology have made our lives better, opening up unimaginable opportunities for growth, development, and knowledge but, at the same time, inevitably also changed our way of being in the world and relating to it. Recovering the human dimension of relationships, physical contact, and real closeness is a powerful antidote against loneliness.

Conclusion

No one can deny the profound connection between diet, health, and happiness. Through this book, based on international-caliber research, we have explored how the Mediterranean diet can significantly enrich our existence, improving both the quality and length of our lives. However, I wish to conclude by broadening our perspective even further. According to the One Health approach, supported by the World Health Organization, human, animal, and environmental health are intrinsically linked. This implies that improving human health not only addresses local health challenges but also significantly contributes to the well-being of our planet.

The Mediterranean diet model, recognized by UNESCO as a World Heritage, stands out for its dual benefit: it improves individual health and it protects the environment. Research has demonstrated its preventive effects on cardiovascular diseases, cancers, and other chronic conditions. From an ecological perspective, it promotes lower consumption of water resources and reduces greenhouse gas emissions compared to diets with a higher intake of meat.

Tim Lang, Professor of Food Policy at City, University of London, argues that "public health goals and ecosystem constraints converge." This means that following a diet beneficial to health also benefits the environment. This has been demonstrated over the years by numerous scientific studies summarized for the first time in 2009 in the "Double Pyramid: food and environmental" created by experts from the BCFN Foundation. This model takes the classic food pyramid, which represents the foods and the proportions they should maintain within a balanced and healthy diet, and adds a new inverted pyramid in which at the tip we have the foods that have the least impact on the environment (based on their ecological footprint) and at the base those that have the highest impact. At first glance, it is evident that foods that are friends of health are also friends of the environment.

Promoting the Mediterranean diet encourages millions of people toward a healthier life and toward responsible and sustainable consumption choices.

Regardless of your personal motivations, whether it's weight loss, protecting your health or your family's health, or if your goal is a larger change concerning your lifestyle and approach to happiness... my wish is that you may pursue a path of health and happiness, and along this journey, leave your mark in a unique and personal way, contributing to an ever-greater well-being project.

THE DOUBLE FOOD AND ENVIRONMENTAL PYRAMID

The Double Pyramid, first developed by the Barilla Center for Food and Nutrition (BCFN) in 2009, emphasizes that food that is good for health is also good for the environment.

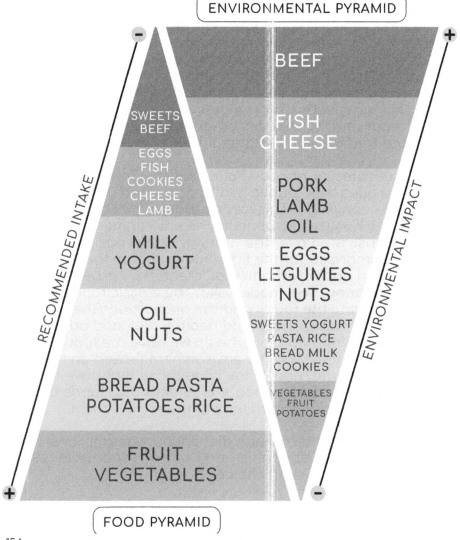

Extra Features

Do you also need to lose weight for your health and well-being?

Often, this is the very reason people become interested in the Mediterranean diet. To complement the general MEAL PLAN in the book, I've created a **weight loss meal plan just for you.**

By following the Mediterranean diet and beginning to change your eating habits, it's natural for those who are overweight to shed a few pounds. However, if you need this to happen more quickly or with certainty, a structured meal plan that helps you accurately manage portions and calories is the best way to proceed.

We've made it easy:

- The Kickstart Meal Plan to Lose Weight is available in two versions to suit different caloric needs—1200 calories and 2000 calories.
- It's flexible: allows members of the same household to enjoy the same dishes, adjusting only the portions, without complicating meal preparations.
- No confusion: All recipes are directly taken from the main book and are marked with the corresponding page number for easy reference.

Are you ready to embrace the Mediterranean way of losing weight?

To get this extra feature, visit **https://bit.ly/MED_LoseWeight** or scan the QR Code below.

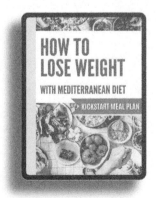

Are you having trouble downloading these contents? Send us an email at info@ heron-books.net. Our support team will be happy to assist you.

References

Dive into the vast body of scientific research that underpins this book and the most distinguished international scientific research. The studies associated with the health benefits of the Mediterranean diet and lifestyle are numerous and constantly evolving; we have gathered them in a carefully curated and regularly updated online database. Through the link, you will have access to the wealth of empirical studies that inspired this book and detail the positive impacts of this diet on various health aspects, enabling you to make more informed dietary and lifestyle decisions based on solid scientific evidence.

To access this resource and deepen your understanding of the empirical benefits of the Mediterranean diet, follow the link or scan the QR code.

https://bit.ly/SCIENCE-BACKED-MEDDIET

About the Author

Dr. Franco Daniele is an Italian-origin nutritionist and longevity medicine researcher, renowned for his expertise in a range of health issues including obesity, celiac disease, diabetes, sports nutrition, metabolic diseases, and eating disorders. His dedication to the field of nutrition and metabolic health is evidenced by his extensive contribution to scientific literature, including scientific reports and review papers, primarily in Italian. His research and outreach focus on chronic disease prevention and weight management, emphasizing the connection between diet and longevity, particularly in Western societies where lifestyle-related diseases are prevalent.

His latest work, "The Science-backed Mediterranean Diet for Beginners," is tailored for a global audience, with a special emphasis on American readers. This choice was inspired by his personal life, as he married a woman from Florida, where he now resides, further fostering his connection to the American public. The book aims to demystify the Mediterranean diet, presenting it as a scientifically sound and accessible lifestyle choice for preventing chronic diseases and managing weight.

Dr. Daniele's writing transcends mere information; it acts as a beacon of empowerment and optimism for those seeking to lead healthier lives. His clear, succinct, and direct approach to writing reflects his belief that the science of nutrition should be accessible to all, especially those most adversely affected by economic disparities or misled by fleeting health trends and misinformation. His latest book encourages readers to save themselves by adopting evidence-based, scientifically-informed lifestyle choices.

With a life split between Florida and Southern Italy, Dr. Daniele enjoys his time with his wife, two children, and close ones, reflecting the very essence of the Mediterranean lifestyle he advocates—a balance of family, health, and sharing.

Conversion Chart

Oven Temperatures

NO FAN	FAN FORCED	FARENHEIT
120 °C	100 °C	250 °C
150 °C	130 °C	300 °C
160 °C	140 °C	325 °C
180 °C	160 °C	350°C
190 °C	170 °C	375°C
200 °C	180 °C	400°C
230 °C	210 °C	450°C
250 °C	230 °C	500°C

Sr Flour = Self Raising

Cup and Spoons

CUP	METRIC
1/4 cup	60 ml
1/3 cup	80 ml
1/2 cup	125ml
1 cup	250 ml
SPOONS	**SPOONS**
1/4 teaspoon	1.25 ml
1/2 teaspoon	2.5 ml
1 teaspoon	5 ml
2 teaspoon	10 ml
1 Tablespoon	20 ml

Liquids

Cup	Metric	Imperial
	30ml	1 fl oz
1/4 Cup	60ml	2 fl oz
1/3 Cup	80 ml	31/2 fl oz
	100 ml	23/4 fl oz
1/2 Cup	125 ml	4 fl oz
	150 ml	5 fl oz
3/4 Cup	180 ml	6 fl oz
	200 ml	7 fl oz
1 Cup	250 ml	83/4 fl oz
11/4 Cups	310 ml	101/2 fl oz
11/2 Cups	375 ml	13 fl oz
13/4 Cups	430 ml	15 fl oz
	475 ml	16 fl oz
2 Cups	500 ml	17 fl oz
21/2 Cups	625 ml	211/2 fl oz
3 Cups	750 ml	26 fl oz
4 Cups	1L	35 fl oz
5 Cups	1.25L	44 fl oz
6 Cups	1.5L	52 fl oz
8 Cups	2L	70 fl oz
10 Cups	2.5L	88 fl oz

Mass

Imperial	Metric
1/4 oz	10g
1/2 oz	15 g
1 oz	30 g
2 oz	60 g
3 oz	90 g
4 oz (1/4 lb)	125 g
5 oz	155 g
6 oz	185 g
7 oz	220 g
8 oz (1/2 lb)	250 g
9 oz	280 g
10 oz	315 g
11 oz	345 g
12 oz (3/4 lb)	375 g
13 oz	410 g
14 oz	440 g
15 oz	470 g
16 oz (1 lb)	500 g
24 oz (11/2 lb)	750 g
32 oz (2 lb)	1kg
48 oz (3 lb)	1.5kg

Made in the USA
Las Vegas, NV
17 July 2024

92404833R00089